W9-CKH-995

Wellness by Design

Wellness by Design

A **ROOM-BY-ROOM** GUIDE TO OPTIMIZING YOUR HOME FOR HEALTH, FITNESS + HAPPINESS

JAMIE GOLD, CKD, CAPS, MCCWC

TILLER PRESS

New York   London   Toronto   Sydney   New Delhi

An Imprint of Simon & Schuster, Inc.
1230 Avenue of the Americas
New York, NY 10020

This publication contains the opinions and ideas of its author.
It is intended to provide helpful and informative material on the subjects addressed in the
publication. It is sold with the understanding that the author and publisher are not engaged in
rendering medical, health, or any other kind of personal professional services in the book.
The reader should consult his or her medical, health, or other competent professional before
adopting any of the suggestions in this book or drawing inferences from it.

The author and publisher specifically disclaim all responsibility for any liability,
loss, or risk, personal or otherwise, that is incurred as a consequence, directly or indirectly,
of the use and application of any of the contents of this book.

First Tiller Press hardcover edition September 2020

TILLER PRESS and colophon are trademarks of Simon & Schuster, Inc.

For information about special discounts for bulk purchases, please
contact Simon & Schuster Special Sales at 1-866-506-1949 or business@simonandschuster.com.

The Simon & Schuster Speakers Bureau can bring authors to your live event.
For more information or to book an event, contact the Simon & Schuster Speakers Bureau
at 1-866-248-3049 or visit our website at www.simonspeakers.com.

Interior design by Jennifer Chung

Manufactured in the United States of America

1   3   5   7   9   10   8   6   4   2

Library of Congress Cataloging-in-Publication Data
Names: Gold, Jamie, 1960– author.
Title: Wellness by design : a room-by-room guide to optimizing your home for health,
fitness, and happiness / by Jamie Gold.
Description: New York : Tiller Press, 2020. | Includes bibliographical references.
Identifiers: LCCN 2020000877 (print) | LCCN 2020000878 (ebook) |
ISBN 9781982139049 (hardcover) | ISBN 9781982139056 (ebook)
Subjects: LCSH: Interior decoration—Health aspects. | Housing and health.
Classification: LCC NK2113 .G644 2020 (print) | LCC NK2113 (ebook) | DDC 747—dc23
LC record available at https://lccn.loc.gov/2020000877
LC ebook record available at https://lccn.loc.gov/2020000878

ISBN 978-1-9821-3904-9
ISBN 978-1-9821-3905-6 (ebook)

This book is dedicated to everyone who believes
they can train, fuel, and accomplish
whatever goals they challenge themselves to achieve . . .

And to my parents, who inspired me
with their example to believe that I could too.

CONTENTS

INTRODUCTION

I bet you picked up this book because you're invested in improving or maintaining your health and you're looking for new ways to do so. That's a great reason. I'm interested in mine, too, and have discovered many connections between where we live and our total well-being, which I look forward to sharing with you in these pages. Let me share a little of my story first—including how I came to learn of these connections, which have already benefited me greatly, and which I believe can benefit you too.

MY STORY

I haven't always been great at taking care of myself. I was reasonably active in my twenties and thirties, swimming, hiking, and strength training after work and on the weekends. But when I finished grad school and started working more demanding jobs in my forties, I began de-stressing with junk food and TV instead of working out or even walking. I became completely sedentary, and the pounds piled on.

When my marriage crashed and burned just before my forty-ninth birthday, I realized that I was a heart attack waiting to happen and needed to get off the dang couch. Fortunately, our subdivision had a heated pool, and I started swimming laps again. I enjoyed both the movement and the calming nature of slicing through the water. I also found that my body started craving healthier foods like fresh fruits and vegetables again to power my laps, a welcome reintroduction to better eating.

That was the start of a three-year journey to losing about a hundred pounds, which I plan to keep off forever! As you may have found yourself, losing lots of weight is much more exciting than maintaining a healthy weight. It elicits compliments from friends, offers new and sleeker wardrobe options, inspires new confidence, and can generate new dating possibilities. Losing weight takes weeks, months, or even a year or more. Maintaining weight takes a lifetime of consistency, long after the thrill has worn off. Many people eventually regain the weight; I've been guilty of a little backsliding too. It's a constant battle as I move toward the big six-oh and beyond.

RETHINKING FITNESS

The most effective strategy for me was changing my mind-set from dieting and exercising to training and fueling. I set a goal: to complete a three-mile Spartan Race in January 2014 after volunteering at a similar event and winning a free entry online. I found an obstacle course racing (OCR) coach in my area, learned how to scale six- and eight-foot walls (not gracefully, mind you!), run trails, and do burpees. Most women in their fifties get their mud at spas; I was getting mine crawling under barbed wire.

After that first OCR event, I set new goals to complete a Spartan Trifecta (5K, 15K, and half-marathon distances in one year), two military-style GoRuck endurance events, two Ragnar trail relays, half and full marathons, and the summiting of Mount Whitney, the highest peak in the lower forty-eight states. Each required dedicated training, proper nutrition, rest, and recovery.

I met other racing, endurance, and mountaineering enthusiasts and joined an active community that loves spending weekends in the mountains, running road and trail races, hiking, and doing all kinds of fun workouts together. We still talk and post about the best foods for performance and avoiding stomach upset during our training sessions and events. We spend nights at each other's homes before race mornings so we'll be closer to the start lines, and we compare recovery strategies for the inevitable injuries and ailments that come from pushing yourself hard. Those strategies often include foam rollers, yoga mats, and the restorative joy of jetted showers and spa tubs.

THE HOME HEALTH CONNECTION

While we may travel to events and work or vacation away from home, most of our fueling and recovery take place where we live. That is true for most everyone, regardless of athletic interests or careers. We meal prep and cook in our kitchens, clean up and unwind in our master bathrooms, and restore our energy in our bedrooms, getting as many hours of sleep as we can before starting our long, busy days.

Our living spaces have a tremendous impact on our physical and emotional well-being, from how they're constructed to how they're organized and decorated. This book explores the many ways they can support or sabotage us, room by room, and shares suggestions for making them healthier, safer, and more functional as we strive to live our best lives. Whether you're renting your first apartment, updating your current house, or building your forever home, you'll find ideas in these pages to improve both your living space and your health.

WELLNESS DESIGN: WHAT'S IN IT FOR YOU?

We have known for a long time that toxic elements in our homes can make us sick. Over the years research findings have led to bans on asbestos and lead as well as limitations on excessive formaldehyde and other indoor pollutants that can impact our indoor air quality. There are many books on the subject of safe building and household materials, but it isn't the only important aspect of wellness design.

There are five facets of wellness design—health and fitness, safety and security, accessibility, functionality, and comfort and joy—and these all contribute to your home's role in your health and well-being. You'll find these facets reflected throughout this book. Let's take a quick look at what they mean for you and the important people in your life.

- FITNESS AND HEALTH covers a broad area, including how your home can help support your exercise goals, nutrition, hygiene, rest, and recovery. It means that your cooking appliances help you prepare healthier meals, and your bedroom is optimized for sleep. It suggests adding steam to your shower for better recovery from illness or injury and to your oven or range for preserving the nutrients in your food. It includes saunas and massaging showerheads for exercise recovery and suggestions for creating workout areas in your living space. *You'll find fitness and health ideas throughout the book.*

- SAFETY AND SECURITY mean that you reduce your chances of experiencing a home disaster. Building codes address many of the major risks, but they don't help if you choose an inexperienced, unlicensed individual to work on your electrical system, for example, or if someone cuts corners during a renovation project that can result in illness or injury. Safety also means having proper ventilation in your kitchen to reduce fire risk and in your bathroom to avoid mold buildup, and having enough task lighting where you cut vegetables to avoid slicing a finger instead of a carrot. Last but definitely not least, safety also relates to security. With so many homes now tied to the Internet through smart-home technology, protecting your privacy and data is an ever-growing challenge, and is definitely tied to your wellness. *You'll find safety and security ideas throughout the book.*

- ACCESSIBILITY means that you, your household members, and your guests can fully enjoy your home unimpeded by injury, illness, disability, or age. It means that you can reach items deep inside your cabinets even if your back is screaming from yesterday's workout; that your partner can shower even if she's on crutches after a rock-climbing fall; and that your grandfather can stay for a holiday weekend even if he's a wheelchair user. Accessibility ensures that you can remain independent and fully able to use your home if or when life's inevitable setbacks occur. *You'll find accessibility-enhancing ideas throughout the book.*

- FUNCTIONALITY means that your home is optimized for peak performance whether you're eating, working, doing chores, or sleeping. A kitchen optimized for functionality makes cleaning up after dinner faster and easier, so you can spend more time relaxing or working out. A more functional kids' bathroom means easier school mornings and pre-bedtime routines, and potentially fewer sick days. An entry area optimized for functionality makes leaving the house less stressful and coming home more pleasant. *You'll find functionality-enhancing ideas throughout the book.*

- COMFORT AND JOY mean that your home is personalized to enhance your emotional and physical well-being. Physical comfort is improved by details like radiant floor heating in your master bath to greet your feet on a wintry day or aromatherapy in your shower to help you de-stress. Joy encompasses the details that accessorize your home, from artwork and memorabilia to area rugs and window coverings. These details can be functional, like doormats, or purely decorative, like family photos.

For example, a beautiful wool area rug warms and softens a tiled living room, but it becomes even better when it's secured in place so that no one trips on a corner. Hanging your race medals on a garage wall welcomes you home with reminders of accomplishments and great times—and that's a mood lifter every time you drive in. Comfort and joy also mean connecting your home with nature. It's been shown that plants purify our air and uplift our mood, and that natural light levels and quality greatly influence our sleep cycles. Additionally, images, fragrances, and sounds of nature can all have health-enhancing benefits. The more your living space connects to nature, and the easier it is for you to access nature outside your doors, the greater potential for improving your well-being. *You'll find comfort and joy ideas throughout the book.*

You may not own your own home at the moment, but that doesn't mean that you don't deserve to have the healthiest living space possible. While some of the ideas in this book won't apply to your current situation, as it generally doesn't make sense to remodel a rental, each chapter has sections titled "Wellness Tips" that apply to renters and homeowners alike, and there are many suggestions related to finishing touches that you can take with you when you move.

The book can help you when you're ready to buy your next—or first—home or if you're a caregiver for a relative who wants to stay in the home where he raised his family. The concepts and suggestions in these pages aren't focused on this year's fad but on time-tested ideas, many rooted in science.

IMPORTANT HEALTH NOTE

Speaking of science, I'm not a health care professional and don't pretend to be one. In fact, one of the important takeaways from the respected Mayo Clinic Wellness Coach Training Program I completed was "Stay in your lane." No one should give advice for which she's not trained or qualified. As a certified coach and wellness design consultant, I take that recommendation seriously and reach out for health care input from a medical specialist whenever I need expertise.

Design professionals will often consult with clients' medical providers about specific needs when they know that someone is under a doctor's care—or recommend that clients talk to their medical team before proceeding with design recommendations, like steam showers or saunas, that can impact their health and safety.

When it comes to health care advice in the pages of this book, I have used direct quotations from experts in their fields (you'll see them under the heading "House Calls" in each of the roomcentric chapters); insights from the many licensed medical professionals I've interviewed through a long career of writing about wellness design for multiple publications; and published consumer advice from respected sources like the Mayo Clinic, Harvard Medical School, the Cleveland Clinic, medical associations, and journals. When I reference "health care professionals" or "medical experts," this is the knowledge base I'm drawing upon.

This book is based on my findings and is not intended to replace consultation with your own health care professional. I wrote *Wellness by Design* to share knowledge about the links between your home and your health from my research and professional experience in the design and wellness fields and from my personal journey from couch potato to midlife weekend warrior with a 2020 training plan and goal to summit Kilimanjaro before I turn sixty.

I encourage you to make your own health care decisions based on your own research and in partnership with a qualified health care provider. And I do hope this book inspires you to set new wellness goals—and help your home live up to them.

What Is **WELLNESS DESIGN?**

If the term "wellness design" is completely new to you, you're not alone. It's a fairly young discipline that has gained acceptance among architects, builders, designers, and remodeling professionals in recent years as we've worked on making healthier places for us all to live and work.

The aim of wellness design is to create a home that works with you every day, including supporting your training regimen, fueling your workouts, and encouraging your recovery afterward, with benefits you may have never considered, like better air quality from non-toxic building materials, pet-friendly features, and high-performance ventilation.

Or perhaps some of the above were among the reasons you chose your home, condo, or apartment in the first place. Maybe you were drawn to the large windows allowing in natural light and views of trees or flowers outside. For many, a chef's kitchen is a huge draw, and you saw yourself creating healthy meals with ease there as soon as you walked in.

Maybe the master bath's spa-style shower reminded you of your resort vacation, and you can definitely see yourself grilling kabobs with your hiking buddies in the outdoor kitchen.

All of these features make a home or apartment community appealing and can influence buying or leasing decisions. They can also enhance the wellness of the people living in them in physical, practical, and emotional ways. Let's take a look at each.

PHYSICAL FEATURES

The physical aspects of wellness design can include anything from a spa-style shower's handheld head with massage setting to help soothe sore muscles after a long run or hike, to the combi steam oven in a fabulous chef's kitchen to help you cook healthier meals. The good news is that you can have both of these features even if you're renting an apartment. *Wellness design is not just for homeowners!*

Physical wellness design features affect breathing, standing and walking, sleeping, cooking, hygiene, working, exercising, and caregiving. From the moment you walk in your door to the moment you leave, your home is supporting (or sabotaging) your well-being in big and small ways.

For example, many fitness-focused adults spend Sunday evenings meal prepping for the week ahead. This can mean several hours spent working in the kitchen. The typical kitchen floor is ceramic tile, a very hard surface that makes extended periods standing on it fatiguing to feet, shins, knees, hips, and back. As a result, it's not uncommon to feel sore after hours of kitchen work, which can be a training issue if you meal prep before your workouts, or a reason to avoid it afterward when you're already tired and achy.

Here's another example: You worked, exercised, showered, ate dinner, and relaxed at home before heading to bed. You're committed to getting at least seven hours of quality sleep on weeknights. Unfortunately, the streetlights outside your bedroom window are blazing through your curtains. It's going to be a long night before another long workday. Blackout panels, shades, or liners will usually solve the problem and aren't terribly expensive to purchase. (Bonus: They can also lower your utility bills.)

There are amenities you can add to every room—from entryway to bedroom to garage—to enhance your home's wellness design quotient, whether you own or rent. Others, like new flooring or a whole-house water filtration system, should be installed by an owner rather than a tenant. Renters can still get their benefits through simple purchases like a cushioned anti-fatigue mat or a faucet-mounted filtration unit.

PRACTICAL FEATURES

No one ever says, "I want to spend more time cleaning my kitchen and bathroom." Appliances, countertops, backsplashes, cabinetry, fixtures, and flooring that are hard to clean may harbor more dirt and germs and definitely take more of your precious time to maintain. That's time you could be spending relaxing or working out. A handful of low-maintenance design and remodeling choices can improve your quality of life, save you time, and create a healthier home.

Another practical feature of wellness design is accessibility, a design term for making it easy to reach and use everything in a space. It's not something that most active, younger adults tend to think about unless they find themselves nursing a sports injury on crutches, trying to get into the back of a vanity cabinet for a heating pad after an Ironman, or caring for a disabled family member. But it's something that older adults, including very active ones, think about often.

Another feature of the chef's kitchen that sold you on your home could be its pantry roll-out trays, the pull-out drawers in every base cabinet, and the swing-out organizer in the corner. These are all accessibility enhancing, and they all also help you to better organize your space for cooking and entertaining.

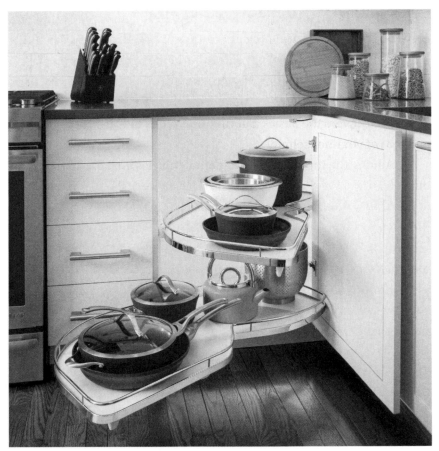

Kitchen organizers make meal prep easier, faster, and more accessible.

Accessibility issues often come up at a home's entrances and in its bathrooms. How easy is it to navigate your way from the curb to your front door, or from your garage to your interior? What if you're heading out for a run with your baby in a jogging stroller or your foot is in a temporary cast? What about your weekend guest whose rugby accident landed him in a wheelchair, or your grandmother visiting with her walker and heavy roller bag?

Accessibility is a physical feature, but it's also a practical one. Making your home more "visitable" (and usable, if you're injured at some point) enhances its wellness potential. (It can also enhance its resale value, as there's a serious shortage of accessible homes in this country.)

WELLNESS TIP
Place a small bench
near your home's
busiest entrance
so that no one has
to juggle packages
while trying to reach
the doorknob or
keys. It serves as
a place to sit for
someone who is
tired or a space
to set things down
for convenience
and balance.

Safety is another practical feature of wellness design. Building codes across the country include mandated smoke detectors, sprinkler systems, carbon monoxide detectors, vent fans for kitchens and bathrooms, and construction standards, so that you can be reasonably certain that your home won't fall down on your head.

That covers the basics, but they don't fully address your safety and that of your household.

Among the top causes of accidental injuries are falls, fires, and burns. (Falls are the leading injury-related cause of death for seniors.) Some of these are preventable, and a home designed for wellness will have slip-resistant flooring materials, anti-scald valves, designer-style grab bars in the tub or shower that blend stylishly with the room's other finishes, as well as a fire extinguisher near the kitchen.

Another way to protect yourself is to avoid hiring unlicensed contractors and tradesmen when you're improving your home, and not buy knockoff remodeling products that might result in mold-causing leaks behind your walls, electrical fires, toxic product fumes, and other hazards. These less expensive products may save you money in the short run but will often cost you far more later when expensive issues develop.

EMOTIONAL FEATURES

Last but definitely not least among wellness design features are those that benefit your emotional health. The place where you live definitely has an emotional component—the difference between a house and a home, you could say. Your home is, or should be, a place of refuge from the outside world. It should welcome you when you walk in the door, and envelop you in comfort while you're inside.

This is especially important in high-stress times, like after a mass shooting, when our screens are filled with violence and chaos. Mental health professionals[1] confirm that watching the news reports that follow these violent events leaves many people—especially teens and young adults—feeling vulnerable, anxious, and fearful, especially if the event happened near where they live. Creating an electronics-free sanctuary at home, where you can meditate, pray, relax, and decompress, helps maintain emotional wellness. It can include a spiritual icon, if faith is part of your life and tradition, or lavender oil diffusers or fabric spray; this flower has been shown to be a mood stabilizer.

Emotional wellness should be part of your home whether you're a tenant or an owner, whether you're staying in a corporate apartment for a month while you work at a client site in another city, or living in the home you've owned with your spouse for forty years. In a temporary or rental setting, you're not going to make permanent changes to the space, but you can bring along a favorite framed photo to sit on the nightstand and greet you in the morning. You can bring a spiritual element to enhance the space, like a prayer rug. You can bring along your favorite throw to wrap yourself in while you watch TV. You can plug in a wireless speaker to play music from your phone or light a candle that reminds you of the pines or jasmine outside your window at home. Scent is the sense with the deepest ties to memory, so bringing fragrances that evoke happy memories or associations create emotional wellness in a temporary or permanent home.

In a house or condo that you own, you can build in even more emotional wellness features. These could be a "man cave" or "she shed," a cozy library with your favorite books, or just a reading or meditation nook in a corner of a bedroom.

Bringing more sunlight into your home is another way to add emotional wellness. Most people are drawn toward rooms filled with natural light. Window sheers that deliver some privacy during the day while allowing more light in is one way to brighten a room. Solar tubes, which are like skylights but easier to install and often less prone to problems, are another way.

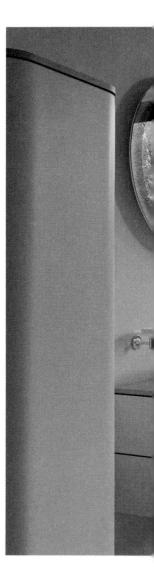

Connecting your indoor spaces with views and access to nature enhances your wellness.

WELLNESS TIP
Add plants in
pots for an easy,
welcoming note and
better indoor air
quality in any room.

Celebrating nature in your home with plants and other natural inspirations—called biophilia—is one more way to add emotional wellness to your space. Plants in particular create a welcoming environment and can help with indoor air quality as well. Natural inspirations can be decorative details like an accent table made of wood from your home state, a water feature that recalls your favorite waterfall hike, or even bird prints that remind you of a recent vacation.

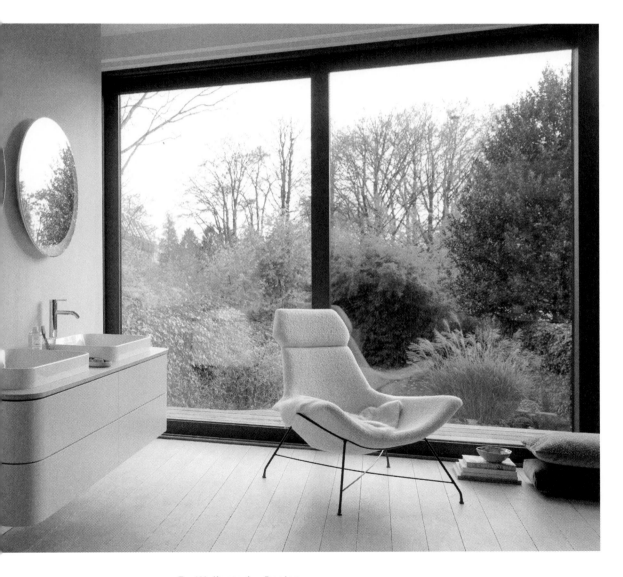

We spend so much time focused on our electronics that connections to nature, both physical (being in a natural environment) and visual (natural light, views, and depictions), can promote stress relief, concentration, healing, and injury recovery, according to medical researchers.[2]

Some homeowners create green walls in their homes' interiors or exteriors. Some cover all or most of the entire vertical surface with edible plants in the kitchen or patio grilling area. Some are purely decorative, as a backdrop to a relaxation space. (You might have seen some of these in hotels, office buildings, or restaurants.) These can be full-wall designs on a balcony or terrace or just an accent feature inside. Green walls vary by space, size, and purpose, but all involve irrigation systems and proper plant selection for your climate. If you're adding a permanent feature to your home, consulting with a horticulturalist who knows which plant species work in your setting and region can be helpful. There are also smaller, freestanding systems that can either be placed on your floor or mounted on a wall. These are smaller investments and can be moved if you rent or plan on relocating.

If you're putting an addition on your home, talk with your architect about maximizing access to natural light. That might mean more or bigger windows or a wall of glass doors that slide all the way open. (Just do it in a way that fits with your home's existing architecture, or the effect will be more jarring than wellness enhancing.)

Decorating with personalized details is wellness design on a smaller scale. These can come from a family photo gallery or be original art that you collected on trips, or a personalized rack with all of your medals that make you smile when you look at them. Rather than buying art that matches your furniture, choose decorative details that match your passions in life, and add a piece to every room where you spend time, including the laundry room and garage. That way you'll have something delightful to look at when you do your least favorite chore or return home tired from a trip.

Buying beautiful organic bedding creates a welcoming bedroom that cradles you in natural fibers and enhances your physical

Green walls can bring nature's wellness benefits and dramatic flair into your living spaces.

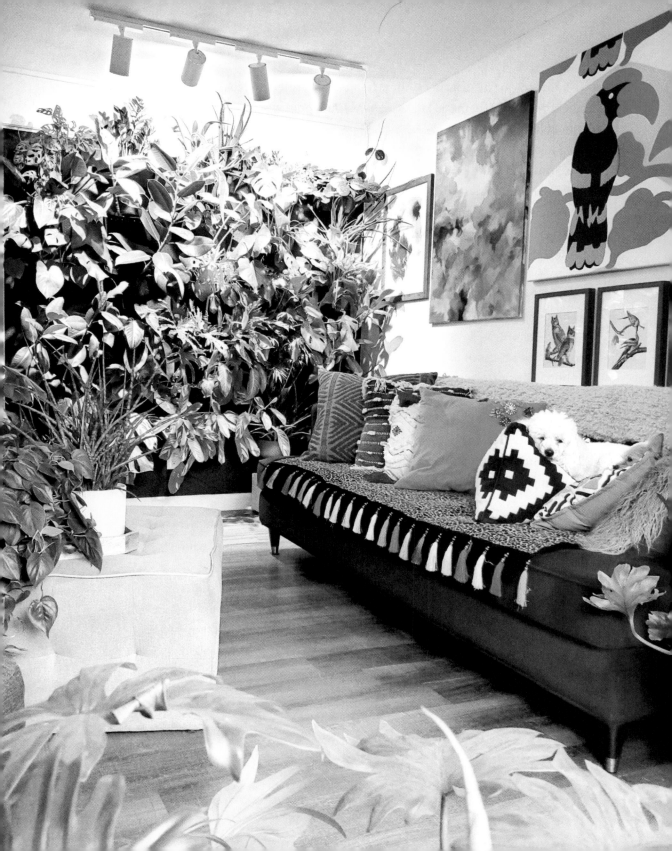

well-being by not off-gassing (industry-speak for releasing toxic fumes from chemical materials or dyes) in the room where you spend the most hours every day.

Plush bath towels give any bathroom a spa touch and feel amazing on your skin, especially fresh off of a towel warmer. Setting your childhood cookie jar on your kitchen counter with energy bars inside instead of Oreos may give you a guilt-free smile and delicious memories. Surround yourself with wellness in every room!

THE BENEFITS OF MINIMALISM

There have been hundreds of articles—and one very popular book and TV series—about the joys of decluttering. Most cover the emotional benefits of clearing out old, broken, and no-longer-loved items from your home, but surprisingly few mention the physical benefits. One or more of these may apply to you or your household:

- Overly cluttered spaces can make it difficult and unsafe to move around in for those who live there, as well as caregivers to older or injured residents, and first responders who need to reach and move occupants in an emergency.
- Too much decoration (or highly reflective surfaces) can be overstimulating for children and for those with autism spectrum issues or dementia.
- Small decorative elements within reach of small hands can become choking hazards.
- Some popular elements, like heavy drapes and throw pillows, can harbor dust mites that can cause allergy or asthma issues for people suffering from those conditions.

This isn't to suggest that you turn your home into a stark, modernist museum. You want to be comfortable and nurtured in your space. Decide which pieces make you and your household members feel great, and donate the rest.

WELLNESS DESIGN OUTSIDE

Wellness design extends beyond your front door. You may not have a patio or yard, but if you're near a park, you're going to get your "nature fix" without a lawn mower. If your neighborhood has bike lanes, you can ride more safely. If your coffeehouse and supermarket are within walking distance, you'll likely walk more.

While there are as yet no established wellness design standards for single family homes, there are standards for multifamily dwellings like apartment communities. These call for features like bike racks, bike paths, and bike share opportunities; community gardens with fruits and vegetables; walking trails and the ability to walk to nearby businesses and services; outdoor fitness equipment and comfortable furniture for socializing; and a smoke-free environment inside and out.

Look for these wellness standards to become more widespread in the U.S. (especially since the government, through Fannie Mae, is now promoting them in its Healthy Housing Rewards initiative). Specific standards for single-family residences will likely follow soon.

In the meantime you can create wellness features in your own home or apartment that work for your needs, interests, space, and budget. We'll be looking at all of these physical, practical, and emotional wellness topics in greater depth throughout this book.

Making Your Whole Home HEALTHIER

Your current home may be the first apartment you rented after college graduation, the dream house you built for your family, or a retirement community condo you're moving into after your kids have flown the nest. Wherever you choose to live, your space should be safe, accessible, and comfortable.

If you're renting, you have less choice, especially in tight rental markets. It may be tempting to go with the first apartment you find, but if the building seems unsafe—if you spot obvious issues like leaks, black mold, or blocked fire exits—you're better off staying with a friend or relative or in a temporary space until you can find a safe place to live.

Fortunately, many apartment, condo, and new-home communities today know that prospective residents are looking for healthy amenities, and the developers and managers of such communities are catering to those interests. This means that the tiny, dark gym of decades ago is now an airy fitness center, possibly with trainers providing classes. Some offer so many options that you can completely drop your health club membership—a boon to your financial wellness too!

START WITH THE RIGHT PROFESSIONAL

If you're buying a resale home, you're going to have a professional, experienced home inspector do a complete inspection before you finalize your sale. You can find someone through a professional inspectors' association website or by referral from someone uninvolved with your home purchase—i.e., someone without a vested interest in your buying the property.

If you're building a home with a custom or production builder, you can also bring in an inspector for a pre-drywall inspection during construction. At this stage in the process, the inspector can easily spot and correct potential hazards like ducting, electrical, and plumbing lines that were improperly installed, preventing problems in years to come.

Whether buying or building, you want to make sure there are no code violations, structural issues, or other problems that can endanger your life or that of someone else in your home, or cost you significant sums to repair later.

Construction specifications are closely regulated, in part to protect a building's occupants in the event of a disaster. We've seen some homes survive major earthquakes and others fall apart in hurricanes. Codes are often strengthened after a natural disaster, so the age of your residence can influence its survivability when the next catastrophe occurs.

If you're building a home, adding on to its size, doing a whole-house remodel, or repairing your residence after a disaster, you're going to want to work with a licensed building professional who keeps current on local and national building codes. It's not uncommon for unlicensed contractors and scammers pretending to be contractors or handymen to roam through damaged neighborhoods in the wake of a storm or temblor, hoping to score quick deposits.

Industry professionals and consumer groups suggest exercising caution when anyone pressures you to start a project, demands full payment, fails to offer a written estimate, asks you to sign a contract with blank spaces, or refuses to provide credentials you can check. It's natural to want to start rebuilding as soon as you can, and substandard operators take advantage of your stress to get you to pay them. Don't fall for it.

Your insurance company or a reputable neighborhood real estate agent can provide an experienced, ethical local professional for your repair. Getting the right person can save you time and money in the long run, whether it's a hurricane rebuild, a room addition, or a remodel. He will also get you through the permitting process quicker, which is reason enough.

This pro could be an architect, an interior designer, a builder, a general contractor, or a design-build firm with architectural designers and contractor talent in-house, depending on the work that needs to be done. Talk to several firms to see which is the best fit, and check not only the clients they provide as references but ask those clients for the contact information of friends who have also used the team you're considering.

Just as the professional you hire should not be the guy in the pickup rolling through your neighborhood after a tornado has turned your block into rubble, your contractor should also not be your nephew's wife's stepfather's best friend who builds houses on the side. (You really don't want anyone who does any significant building work on the side.)

The professionals you work with should have their required licenses in good standing. You can check on these on your state's licensing board website. You can also check on complaints against them with the Better Business Bureau. Online ratings aren't always reliable, so when you're investing tens or hundreds of thousands of dollars in a major home project, it's worth it to do some extra checking. In the end, your peace of mind will be worth it.

Let's say you're going to do the work yourself; many people do these days. It's not a bad idea to consult with a professional first to see if the plans and ideas you're considering are sound. It might cost you time and money to get such a review, but making a dangerous mistake because you don't know or have overlooked something important could cost you more.

YOUR HOME'S COMPONENTS

Whether you're living in an apartment or a single-family house, your home has mechanical systems that make it habitable. These include the ventilation, plumbing, electrical, and heating and cooling systems. If any of these stops working properly, you're going to need to have it fixed pretty quickly or be uncomfortable, inconvenienced, and possibly endangered. If you're a tenant, you get to call the landlord and hope the response is quick. If you're a homeowner, this becomes one more project for you to handle.

Beyond operating properly, there are enhancements available to make each system more health enhancing. If you're building or remodeling, they're worth knowing about and considering.

Ventilation

The air inside your home may be more polluted than the air outside, especially if your home is newer. As builders have increased the energy efficiency of homes, they've reduced the opportunities for bad air to escape. This means fumes you may not be aware of—from carpeting, paint, cabinetry, furniture, electronics, and household cleaning products—can stay trapped in your living spaces. Poor indoor air quality is considered to be a major health hazard by the Environmental Protection Agency, especially since we spend up to 90 percent of our time indoors.

The fact that there are so many more chemicals in our homes' building products than there were in earlier generations hasn't helped, either. That carpet protectant that keeps pet stains at bay can be emitting carcinogens long after you move in.

If you're buying a home, you can have the air tested for allergens, toxins, and other issues that can impact your health. An environmental consultant or air quality testing professional can advise you on what might be in your home—especially if a family member has been having breathing issues or other reactions since moving in—and how to remedy the problem. You can also install carbon monoxide, radon, and other air quality monitors that will alert you to problems.

Air quality monitors alert you to otherwise undetectable dangers in your home, such as radon.

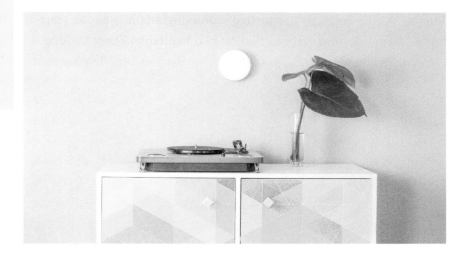

If you're building a home, you can work with a green building professional to avoid the use of toxic materials in your project. This is especially beneficial for those who have existing health issues or known sensitivities that can be made worse by chemical exposure.

Plumbing

Some municipal water systems are better than others. Unless you're on a well, you're getting your water from one of them and are subject to its quality. There can also be issues with well water, depending on where you're living. While many homeowners install kitchen sink filters or use filtered water from their refrigerators for drinking, that doesn't address the water quality in your bathroom sinks, where you and your family might take vitamins and medicine, brush your teeth, and wash your faces. It also doesn't address the water quality in your shower, which can impact the health of your skin and hair.

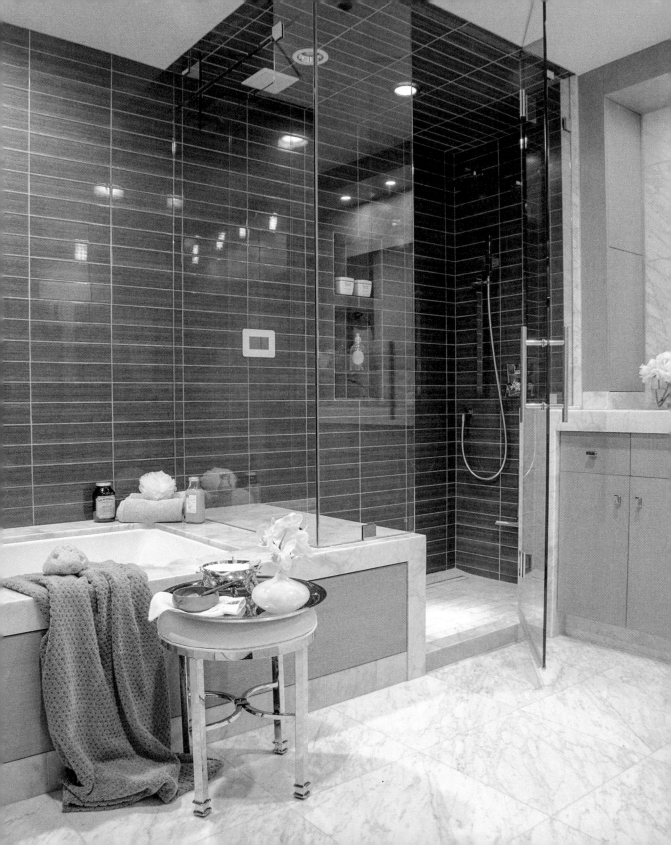

A whole-house water filtration system can improve the quality of all of the water that comes into your home by filtering it at the entry point. Its main drawback is its expense, which may put it out of reach of some households. If you're in a development or condo building, you may be able to negotiate a better rate together with your neighbors. If the system comes with a leak detector, as some do, you may also be able to negotiate a reduction to your homeowner insurance policy.

Leak detectors are beneficial on their own as well, and you can find one through several manufacturers. They can alert your smartphone to a problem and even shut off the water if there's a leak. This can save you a lot of stress and money if you're traveling when a problem occurs or if you have a second home. It's worth asking your insurance company whether they offer a discount for this type of system. Even if they don't, the cost of the system can be less than your deductible and prevent the kind of plumbing issues that can suck up funds you'd much rather spend on your next vacation.

Electrical

Modern homes built to code will have safe electrical systems with proper grounding and circuit breakers. That's the good news. The bad news is the proliferation of devices, gadgets, electronics, and small appliances that so many of us use. Too many house fires start with overloaded, poorly made, or pet-damaged extension cords.

A surge protector can help prevent a house fire and damage to your equipment, and should be used in place of a power strip without one. A heat-producing appliance should never be used with an extension cord. Have a licensed electrician add an outlet if you need one.

There are many reasons to add outlets to your home even if you're not doing a full-scale remodeling project. One is the addition of a charging station in the spot that's most convenient for you to power up your phone, tablet, or both. Another common reason for adding an outlet is the replacement of a standard toilet for one with bidet functionality. In that case, the electrician will place one in close

Water filtration enhances the many benefits steam showers provide.

proximity to the fixture, a spot where builders haven't traditionally included outlets. (They may start soon as bidet features become more popular; many designers already suggest including them when you build or remodel.)

Tied in with your electrical system is your home's lighting. Depending on where you live and the region's building codes, your light fixtures could be using compact fluorescent light bulbs (CFLs) or light-emitting diodes (LEDs) to meet energy efficiency requirements. LEDs are becoming the more popular standard because of their energy savings, but their blue light can impact sleep cycles. (So can the light from your cell phone or tablet screen, for that matter.)

LEDs also offer the advantage of excellent longevity. That means you may not have to replace the recessed-ceiling light bulb for a decade or more, and staying off a ladder to change it eliminates one potential injury. This is particularly beneficial if the person who'd otherwise be doing the replacement is someone with balance issues, like your elderly father-in-law.

There is disagreement in the medical community about the health effects of CFLs. Some believe that the flicker you may not even perceive could still impact your stress levels. Others believe there's no effect at all. If you're finding that you get headaches or feel poorly when you're in a room lit by CFLs, try replacing those bulbs with LEDs and see if you feel better. (Be very careful not to break the bulbs when disposing of them!)

New LED lighting systems, often called humancentric or circadian, seek to solve the blue-light sleep deprivation issue by mimicking the sun's natural lighting cycle through the day. They are typically tied in with a smart home system so that the homeowner doesn't need to do anything to get the benefit. You may want to consult with a smart home professional to personalize to your needs; we don't all share the same body clock.

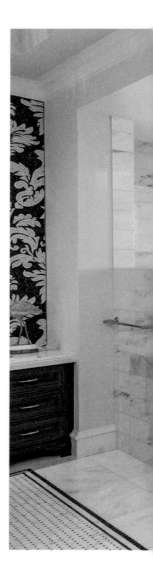

Humancentric (also called circadian) lighting is helpful for getting more and better sleep.

HEATING AND COOLING SYSTEMS

Many modern homes have central air conditioning and forced-air heat. These systems need to be properly sized and well maintained to do their job well and ensure your indoor air quality. If you're a home-owner, you'll be calling in an HVAC professional to do this installation for you.

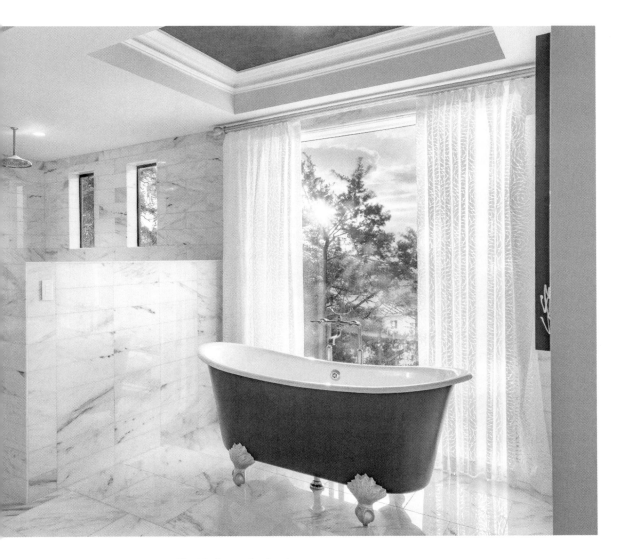

You can also use special HEPA filters with your system to improve your home's indoor air quality. This is especially helpful for allergy and asthma sufferers because these filters trap pollen, pet dander, cigarette smoke, and dust mites so that you or an affected family member don't have to breathe them.

If you're in a region of the country with a temperate climate and good air quality, keeping your windows open can also improve your indoor comfort and health.

Another heating option to consider is a fireplace. For many people, fireplaces evoke romance, comfort, and nostalgia. There are a few options you can choose for these warming features. A wood-burning fireplace is the most authentic with its crackle and roar. You may even enjoy the opportunity to gather your own wood on local hikes and chop it when you get home. (Both can be great workouts!) In some regions, however, wood-burning models are banned because of air pollution considerations. If that's not the case where you live, you can enjoy yours, but be sure to do so safely! Ensure that your chimney is clear, your damper open, your flue clean, and your fireplace inspected before using it for the first time (especially if you just moved into a resale home). Your fireplace should have a screen and doors. You should also have a set of fireplace tools handy so you don't have to move logs with your hands and you can scoop out ash between uses.

Gas fireplaces are more convenient, as you can generally just flip a switch to turn them on. These, too, should have doors to keep children or pets from getting burned. Ventless gas fireplaces are appealing to some, because they can be installed without chimneys and are thus remodel-friendly; but they do vent into the room, which is less than ideal, and are not allowed in all states at this time.

Both gas and wood fireplaces require regular maintenance to continue operating safely. Both should also be professionally inspected annually and call for having fire extinguishers and carbon monoxide detectors nearby.

Another convenient alternative is an electric fireplace, which

WELLNESS TIP
Opening your windows for even five or ten minutes a day can let stale odors escape and enhance your mood with the sounds of nature.

won't send fumes or sparks into your home and are generally kid- and pet-safe. However, even though they can warm a smaller room, most don't offer the realistic flames of wood or even gas models.

PROBLEM-SOLVING AND PROBLEM AVOIDANCE

If one of the systems in your home fails, you're going to have to deal with it to maintain your qualify of life. If you're renting an apartment or house, as noted above, contact the owner or property management company to remedy the situation. It's in their best interest to solve problems before they become larger and more expensive to fix. Hopefully, that applies to your living situation. (Tenant advocacy groups or your city council member can potentially help if your landlord's representatives won't resolve unsafe living conditions.)

Homeowners are best off contacting a recommended, licensed professional, from an HVAC professional for heating, cooling, or ventilation issues to a plumber or electrician to address problems in those systems. You might save money in the short term by bringing in an unlicensed handyman, but if he misses bigger issues, that will cost you more in the long run.

If you're planning on building a home, completing a remodel, or adding on to your house, you'll be choosing components with your building professional. It's often tempting to economize, especially on the components you don't see. But when it comes to your home's systems, a penny saved in the build can result in many dollars expended down the line.

Here's a simple example: You love the style of a European shower system, but not its hefty price tag. You find a knockoff online with the same looks, but it costs considerably less. There are reasons why: it's made from inferior materials, its assembly was not properly supervised, and its valve doesn't have the same quality engineering that the European model has. You buy it anyway, and have your plumber install it behind your shower surround.

A few years later—after the warranty has expired, of course—it starts leaking behind the shower wall. Your savings go down the drain with the wasted water, and you have to hire a professional to repair the damage and replace the faulty parts. If you were lucky, you were home when this started to happen, you noticed it quickly, and you didn't have to deal with nasty mold growth in your bathroom.

What does all of this have to do with wellness? First, a poorly constructed home can risk your safety and life if there's a natural disaster it won't withstand. For example, Hurricane Andrew took sixty-six lives (directly and indirectly), destroyed more than twenty-five thousand homes, and damaged more than one hundred thousand others. It also led to improved building codes—and more stringent code enforcement—to reduce loss of life and property from future storms. That means greater safety and peace of mind for residents in hurricane zones.

Second, a home built with potentially dangerous building products can risk the health of its occupants, and you may not know until an issue arises. Take, for instance, the mass quantity of defective drywall imported in the United States and Canada during the prerecession housing boom. (Sadly, that included drywall used to repair homes after Hurricane Katrina.)

These poorly made wall surfaces off-gassed toxic fumes into the interiors they were used for, creating breathing issues, headaches, and other health problems for residents. They also damaged the home's wiring and expensive appliances and electronics plugged into it. Beyond the health issues were the immense stresses caused by having to move out of these homes and deal with lawsuits.

You can't avoid every hazard in life, unfortunately, but you can take certain precautions to reduce your chances of being the victim of an inferior home product or construction. If you're looking for a rental, bring your fellow tenants before signing a lease. If someone who will be living there experiences physical discomfort when entering the space, you'll want to look elsewhere.

If you're going to buy a home, you can have an air quality inspection along with a standard home inspection. This can be especially helpful if someone moving in has allergies or respiratory issues. If you're building or remodeling, you can avoid products that off-gas, knockoffs that won't stand the test of time, and construction people who aren't licensed. Peace of mind is a definite wellness benefit.

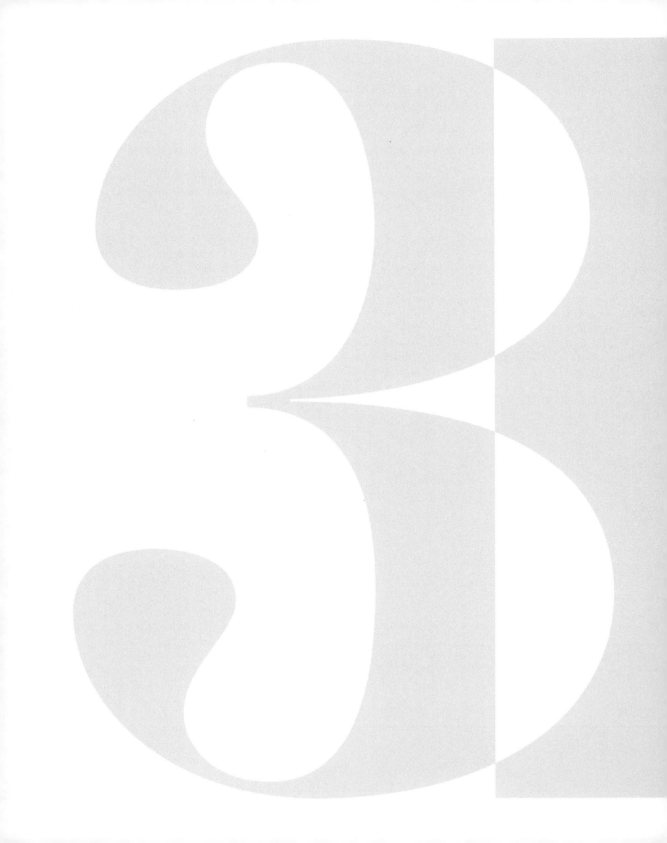

MATERIAL CHOICES

I f you've ever remodeled a room or built a home, you have some idea how many decisions are involved. The fun ones include choosing colors, design accents, and accessories. The more consequential—and sometimes challenging— choices involve selecting the materials you'll incorporate into the space.

These range from floors to cabinetry to countertops to fabrics and wall coverings. These are not just style choices, you'll soon realize. What you pick will determine how a surface feels, how it wears, what maintenance it requires, and how it can impact your health and that of others in your household.

The wrong choice can mean extra hours spent working to keep a countertop, seat cushions, or cabinet fronts looking like new; preventing your baby from breathing carpet fumes when she crawls across the room; or alleviating your partner's aching joints after standing for long hours meal prepping on a painfully hard floor.

Chances are, you're not aware of these potential issues when you fall in love with a glossy, soft, or superhard surface. Let's take a look at some wellness options in each category, along with their pros and cons.

CERAMIC AND PORCELAIN

These materials have proven wellness benefits: They're low-maintenance and generally nontoxic when they come from a known source like the United States, Spain, or Italy—nations with strong certification standards against lead glaze content. (If you're not sure, research the brand before buying. You can do this by requesting a specification sheet or the safety data sheet, or SDS.)

Ceramic and porcelain won't trigger allergies or respiratory issues, as they don't off-gas or trap dust mites, pet dander, or other indoor pollutants. They're also durable, stylistically versatile, and moisture-resistant. Both are made from clay materials fired at extremely high temperatures.

Porcelain is harder and more water-resistant than ceramic, making it a good choice for outdoor living areas and tub/shower spaces in particular, although you'll want to add slip resistance for flooring in both of these applications. Because of its superior hardness, porcelain is a better choice for flooring overall, as ceramic can crack more easily. (Ceramic is popular for affordable wall tiles, where it's lighter and easier to install, but is used as flooring in many older homes.)

Slip resistance can be beneficial on kitchen and entryway floors, too, especially for households with active children or seniors. These are spaces that are more prone toward exposure to water, like spills in the kitchen and rain tracked into an entry. The less slickness, the less chance of someone slipping and falling on it. For safe slip resistance, your tile should have a dynamic coefficient of friction (DCOF) of greater than 0.42; you can find this in the manufacturer's specifications.

Some porcelain is rated as "through body," which means the top finish extends through the body of the tile; if it's chipped, it won't show the damage as readily as its ceramic or non-through-body counterparts. When installed with minimal grout lines—usually requiring rectified porcelain tile—it's even lower-maintenance. Less grout means less time spent scrubbing grape juice spilled by your child or tomato sauce splashed while cooking.

WELLNESS TIP
If you're not in a
position to change
the flooring in your
kitchen, add an anti-
fatigue mat to the
space where you
stand the longest.

Porcelain tiles are ideal for installation over radiant heat flooring systems. These are popular for kitchens, full bathrooms, and even
outdoor living spaces. Unlike its natural stone counterparts—e.g.,
marble or granite—it never needs to be sealed, eliminating one time-
consuming chore from your schedule. New manufacturing technologies
create finishes that can realistically reproduce marble, granite, and
exotic stones. It can also mimic the look of wood in spaces like outdoor
living areas and full bathrooms that aren't ideal for wood's moisture
sensitivity.

In many porcelain lines, it is possible to select slip-resistant outdoor tile to install next to its matching indoor counterpart on the other
side of a wall or door. This helps create a worry-free indoor-outdoor
living area you can enjoy for years to come.

The one wellness negative for tile is its hardness when used
for flooring. This can make falls more painful, and standing on it for
extended periods—while meal prepping or using a standing desk, for
example—can create back, hip, knee, and foot strain. There are mitigat-
ing measures that you can take, though. A soft rug or bath mat held in
place with anti-slip devices can cushion falls in the bathroom, and an
anti-fatigue mat can relieve soreness from standing for long periods.

New porcelain formats include oversized slabs that are ideal for
countertops and shower surrounds. When used as countertops, they
create a low-maintenance and durable surface for your kitchen, bathroom, or outdoor living space. Porcelain can handle direct sunlight
and frost, and is a nonporous material, important for food preparation.
These slabs can also be shaped into an integral sink, creating a low-
maintenance vanity area or kitchen workstation, and several brands
are offering countertops with built-in induction burners, creating an
easy-to-clean, super-sleek surface.

When used for shower surrounds, porcelain slabs require minimal grout (just for corners) and are super-easy to maintain. Less grout
means less opportunity for kitchen staining or shower mildew.

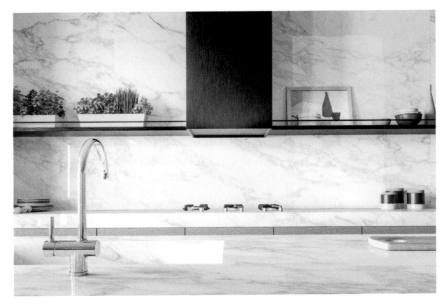

Porcelain, long used for floor and wall tiling, is increasingly being used for durable, family-friendly countertops and cabinet cladding.

Porcelain is being used for cabinet fronts now, too, and makes an excellent alternative to traditional materials like wood and laminate. This creates a contemporary look that is also extremely durable, moisture-resistant, and easy to clean. (If you're considering a refacing project with these fronts, you'll also need new hinges designed for thinner doors.)

WOOD AND BAMBOO

Wood is a popular material for flooring, cabinetry, countertops, and even wall and ceiling coverings. Much of what's sold today for floors, walls, and cabinets is engineered, with a layer of factory-finished wood veneer protected by sealers and glued to an unfinished backing material. For floors, that's usually plywood. For cabinets, it's typically either plywood or compressed wood composites like particleboard or medium-density fiberboard (MDF).

Engineered wood floors are fairly durable and low-maintenance. When safely low in formaldehyde content—meaning they are made without urea-formaldehyde (UF) glues—they're good for allergy sufferers and those with respiratory issues. It's not uncommon for homeowners to address those health issues by tearing out carpeting in favor of wood. Because they float over a moisture-blocking underlay, engineered wood floors are sometimes considered "spongy." That may not appeal to wood purists, but it can be more comfortable to stand on for longer periods.

Homeowners concerned about sustainability sometimes choose renewable bamboo flooring as an alternative to engineered wood. While it is installed the same way, much of the bamboo flooring available today is manufactured overseas and may contain toxic adhesives and formaldehyde. You can find certified bamboo to help reduce these risks. High-quality bamboo flooring will wear as well as wood; less expensive planks are more prone to scratching and denting—something to consider if you have large dogs or active children. Bamboo is a good choice for areas that can experience spills, like kitchen floors, as it is less likely than wood to be damaged by them. It can also work in a powder room but not necessarily in a full bathroom with a tub or shower.

Cabinets made with pressed wood panels should either be no-added-formaldehyde or ultralow-off-gassing formaldehyde. There are wood cabinet options with completely nontoxic finishes and construction. These tend to be custom and more expensive, but if someone in your household is extremely sensitive to chemical exposure, it can be worth the investment to avoid discomfort and potential medical bills.

If you're considering wood paneling, wainscoting, beadboard, shiplap, or wood ceiling cladding, you should ensure that your selection does not include excessive formaldehyde, either, just as you would with cabinetry.

Wood is also popular for countertops ranging from utilitarian butcher block to beautiful premium walnut. If you're using it for your kitchen prep area, rather than just as a decorative breakfast bar or powder room countertop, you're going to need an oil-finished slab, and

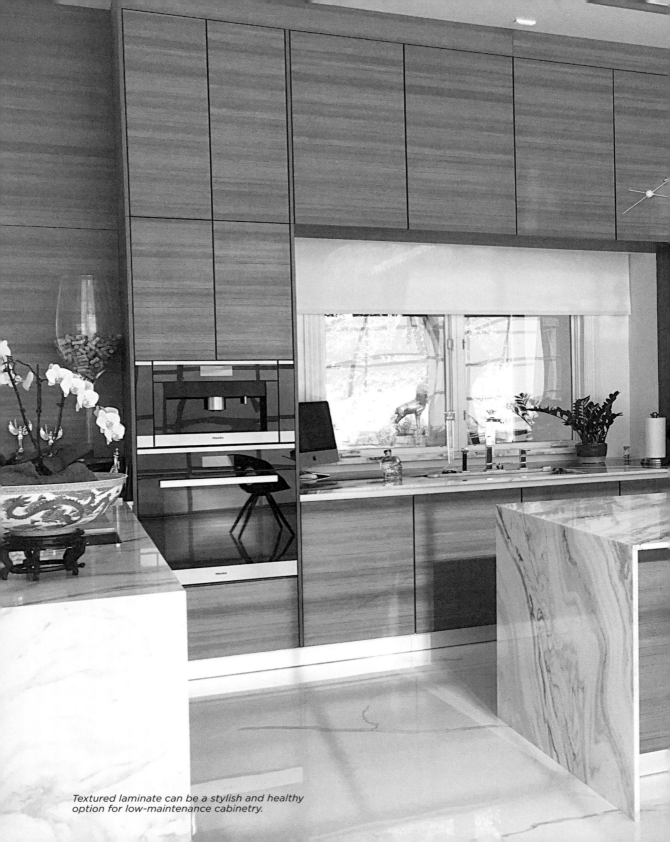

Textured laminate can be a stylish and healthy option for low-maintenance cabinetry.

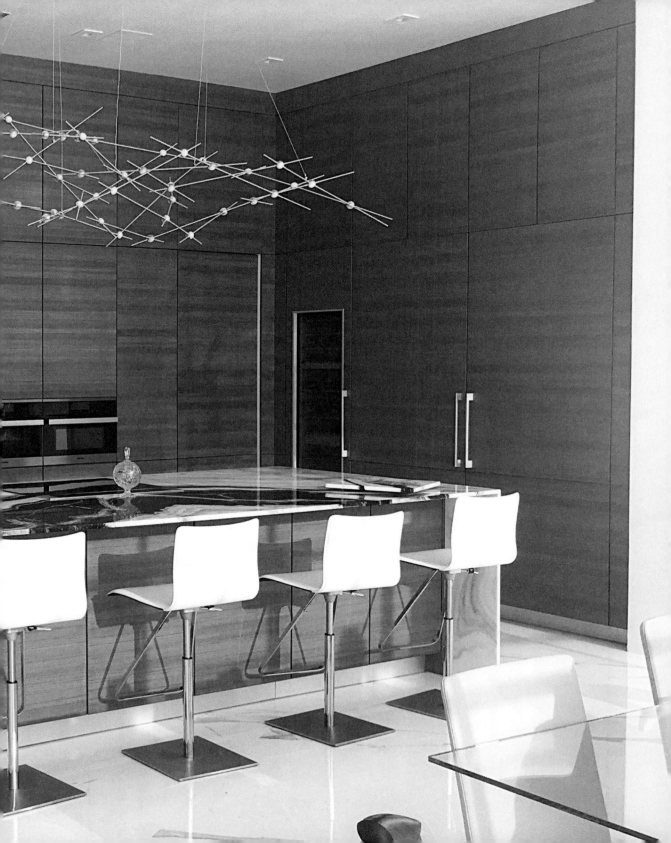

it will require regular maintenance. Think about whether you want to invest that time before opting for wood prep surfacing.

LAMINATE AND VINYL

Laminate and vinyl, often called luxury vinyl tile (LVT), are also often chosen as wood floor alternatives, because they look like wood but cost less. Like bamboo, laminate and LVT can include dangerous levels of chemical toxins (formaldehyde in laminate and phthalates in vinyl). Look for eco-certified planks in both categories to reduce your risk of indoor air pollution.

Laminate and LVT planks cannot be refinished, so they are less worry-free than wood—something to consider in a busy household— but they are fairly durable. Laminate flooring does tend to show scratches that cannot be buffed out, so this should be considered if your favorite hiking buddy and roommate is a large, active dog.

Phthalate-free LVT does have two wellness benefits: It's soft underfoot, making it a good option for children's and senior's spaces and for any rooms where you spend hours standing, and it's low-maintenance. While marketed as water-resistant for kitchens and bathrooms, some tests have shown damaging penetration. Placing LVT in a room with a heavy concentration of water, like a kids' bath, for example, may not be a great long-term solution.

In addition to flooring, laminate is also used for countertops and cabinet fronts. Laminate countertops tend to be fairly afford-able and easy to clean. However, they are easily damaged and non-repairable. You'll typically find them in older starter homes and inexpensive rentals.

Laminate cabinet fronts, on the other hand, have come a long way in durability (and style). They come in gloss or textured finishes. Like more expensive wood lacquer and lustrous MDF finished panels, the gloss is generally more prone to showing fingerprints, and thus higher-maintenance. The textured finishes are often made to look like wood, but they show less and clean up more easily. As with laminate floors (and MDF), you'll want to make sure your laminate-front cabinets are made without harmful formaldehyde.

METAL

Metal may not be the first material to leap to mind when it comes to cabinetry or countertops, but it has some wellness benefits to offer for both. Metal's hygienic properties make it a top choice for restaurant and hospital kitchens. If you're choosing stainless steel countertops, you don't have to worry about foodborne contaminants seeping into its surface, and it is extremely low-maintenance and heat-resistant. That makes it a durable option for a well-used kitchen. On the flip side, it can also make for a noisy kitchen, and the lower-quality, higher-gauge versions dent and scratch fairly easily.

Stainless steel sinks are also extremely durable and low-maintenance. As with countertops, the lower the gauge, the better the material. Properly cared for, a 16- or 18-gauge stainless steel sink should serve you well for decades.

Copper is also used for sinks and countertops, both in the kitchen and bathroom, and is easy to maintain if you're comfortable with its naturally changing color over time. One of its benefits for kitchen prep areas is its natural antibacterial properties. If you seal the top to maintain its warm red finish, you'll defeat this property. Sealed countertops also require periodic treatment.

Zinc is also an antimicrobial metal that can work for kitchen spaces, but it is not very heat- or stain-resistant. If you use trivets and cutting boards and you like a natural patina, it can be a good option for a prep island top.

Metal cabinets aren't as popular for indoor kitchens today as they were decades ago, when a colorful mid-century kitchen might sport glossy crayon-hued cabinetry. Homeowners liked their style and easy-wipe fronts. You may still find some in vintage or retro-style homes.

Rather than seeking out metal cabinets, you may opt to include some open metal shelving for your kitchen. That can be a freestanding rack along the lines of what you'd find in a restaurant kitchen if you want an industrial look, instant visibility, and easy access. Or you can opt for wall-mounted stainless steel shelves in place of cabinets. This also offers easy access and visibility. However, both options expose their contents to more potential breakage and kitchen soiling than closed cabinetry.

The more common applications for metal cabinetry today are outdoors and in garages. Stainless steel cabinets can provide the foundation for a low-maintenance, durable outdoor kitchen, especially when powder coated, which won't show fingerprints as readily. Steel garage cabinets tend to be sturdy and durable, but their finish can be damaged by exposure to corrosive chemicals.

QUARTZ, MINERAL AND HYBRID

Quartz countertops, also referred to as engineered stone and sold under brand names like Silestone, Cambria, and Caesarstone, have emerged as a popular alternative to granite. Like that natural stone, quartz is extremely heat- and scratch-resistant, making it a durable surface for high-traffic spaces like kitchens. Unlike granite, however, engineered stone is nonporous and never needs to be sealed. It's extremely stain-resistant, so you don't need to worry if you spill a glass of wine or if acidic lemon juice lands on it. Wipe off your quartz counter in a reasonable amount of time and it should be just fine.

It does have two small disadvantages. First, most can't be used outdoors, so you'll need an alternative material for your outdoor kitchen. Second, given its hardness (like granite's), someone with depth perception issues might find himself with bruises if he bumps into it, and you can end up with broken drinking glasses from setting them down too roughly on the surface.

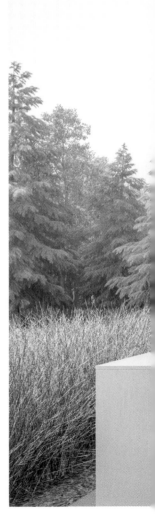

Innovative new materials make outdoor entertaining easier and healthier.

There is a new quartz hybrid product known by the brand name Dekton by Cosentino that combines quartz and porcelain. It blends quartz's heat, scratch, and stain resistance with porcelain's suitability for outdoor use.

Geoluxe is another new, durable, low-maintenance product that's appropriate for indoor or outdoor surfaces. It's a compressed

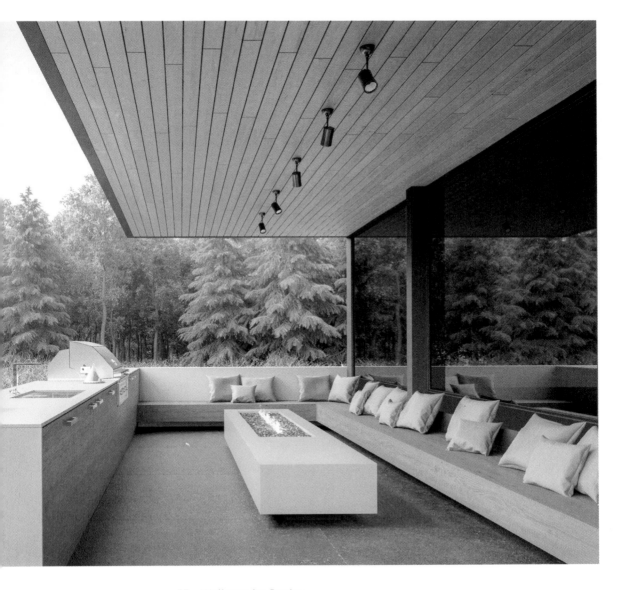

natural mineral that is similar to quartz in appearance but rated for exterior use. Like porcelain, it can accept built-in induction hobs and be used in place of tile on floors and walls.

Another interesting hybrid is Fenix NTM, which blends a solid surface and laminate in a low-maintenance, repairable finish. It's being used for countertops, furniture, and cabinetry surfacing. The touch is soft and matte, making it an appealing, easy-to-care-for material for interior uses.

SOLID SURFACE

"Solid surface" is the generic term for man-made surfaces commonly used for tubs, shower stalls, sinks, and countertops. They are made of acrylic, polyester resins, and other blended materials. The composition varies by manufacturer.

Solid surface is usually a low-sheen surface and is consistently nonporous and germ-, stain-, and mildew-resistant. These properties make it a popular choice for hospitals and other clinical environments and for low-maintenance home interiors. It is not rated or warranted for outdoor use.

When used for countertops, solid surface gives a seamless appearance and can be paired with an integral solid surface sink. Without exposed edges to clean, these sinks are easy to maintain and keep germ-free.

Popular brand names for solid surface countertops include Corian and LG Hausys Hi-Macs, but solid surface is also the material used for many freestanding bathtubs, cultured marble vanity tops, and shower surrounds. These are often sold under less familiar brand names, ranging from affordable builder-grade materials to premium trophy tubs.

Solid surface is fairly easy to scratch or ding, but minor surface damage can usually be buffed out with a minor abrasive. (Check your owner's manual if you purchased it yourself, or go with the least abrasive scouring pad or lowest-grit sandpaper if you're not sure of the brand.) If you damage your solid surface countertop beyond a small DIY project, it can usually be professionally repaired.

CORK

Cork is a natural material most often used for flooring. One of its great wellness benefits is its softness. This is a surface that is easy to stand on for long periods of time, making it ideal for kitchens, hobby rooms, and standing desk areas. It can also cover the floors most often used by an older resident with balance issues or in children's rooms. Another wellness benefit of cork is that it's naturally hypoallergenic and anti-microbial, improving your indoor air quality and helping household members with environmental sensitivities.

On the downside, it is susceptible to fading in direct sunlight, scratching, puncturing, dings, and dents, and some of the more afford-able products—usually agglomerated, particleboard equivalent for cork—need to be sealed; check before you buy! If you're uncomfortable with imperfections, this may not be the surface for you.

LINOLEUM

This flooring material, made from natural materials like linseed oil (from which its name derives) and flax, is more than a century old. Your grandmother's kitchen may have had linoleum floors! Many people confuse it with vinyl, but they are very different surfaces; vinyl is an engineered product that can off-gas. (If you're choosing vinyl—often referred to as resilient flooring—choose phthalate-free products without postconsumer recycled content, as noted earlier.)

Like cork, linoleum is antimicrobial, hypoallergenic, and fairly soft to stand on for long spells. However, it is much more moisture-resistant and harder to damage than cork. It is easy to clean and extremely durable.

If you opt for linoleum tiles rather than sheet material, you can pop out a tile if one does happen to get damaged. You can also create very personalized style with tile patterns, if that's something your creative soul calls for! It's a great surface for game rooms or an authentic retro kitchen redo.

On the downside, this flooring can darken if not treated with a factory coating, and can be damaged by contact with sharp objects. While moisture-resistant, it's not ideal for high-humidity spaces like full bathrooms.

RUBBER

Another antimicrobial, hypoallergenic flooring material is rubber. It is durable but soft underfoot and generally low-maintenance, making it a good option for home gyms, laundry rooms, play areas, and other heavily used spaces. Like cork and linoleum, rubber also muffles sound.

One downside can be its distinctive smell, strongest when new and natural rather than synthetic rubber. On the other hand, synthetic rubber can off-gas if burned; avoid postconsumer recycled crumb rubber. It can also be slippery when wet, and some products, like oil, can stain it. That makes it less than ideal for kitchen or garage flooring. Consider rubber for playrooms and home gyms.

WOOL

Some people love the softness and warmth of carpeting, especially in bedrooms. Unfortunately, much of what's available today is treated with chemicals for stain protection that can off-gas. Even their backing materials can be hazardous if they contain vinyl, polyurethane, or fly ash.

A more natural albeit expensive alternative is wool. Wool is naturally dirt-repellent, hypoallergenic (for those without wool-specific allergies), and flame retardant, and can be made without chemicals.

Note that there are brands that use chemical dyes and anti-insect protectants that may affect those with sensitivities; check before you buy.

Natural wool is also a good bedding option. It is hypoallergenic (again, for those without wool allergies), will resist dust mites, and is naturally temperature regulating. (Hikers love wearing wool layers for that reason.)

Wool's biggest negative is cost, but if you're buying, decorating, building, or remodeling for long-term use, it will likely pay for itself with its longevity.

There are additional materials that are ideal for outdoor use. You'll find those described in chapter 6, "Outdoor Living Spaces."

Smart Home TECHNOLOGY

You've probably noticed that technology is showing up in almost every area of our lives, including our health and wellness. We track our runs on sports watches, monitor our calories and connect with our doctors on smartphone apps, and share workout tips and healthy recipes with friends on social media. Perhaps you're also asking a voice assistant like Alexa or Google Home to play your favorite exercise jams or share a weather report for your weekend hiking trip.

If you're buying a recently constructed home—or building one yourself—you're likely getting a suite of smart home features. What are their benefits and drawbacks as far as your health and well-being? It's not a simple, one-size-fits-all answer, but it's essential to know what's available and how it can impact your life so you can equip your home in a way that makes sense for you and your family.

SECURITY

One of the most popular smart home applications is security. This can range from a video doorbell that lets you see who's approaching your entrance remotely (or who stole your cleats from your porch) to digital door locks that provide a separate code for each household member and anyone who may need access to your home while you're away, like a pet sitter. (If you change sitters, you can delete the code more easily than getting your locks rekeyed.)

The digital entry systems can keep you or your child from being locked out if a key is lost or misplaced, adding an element of safety. It can also let you know if your teens made it home from school or practice, or if the dog walker showed up as scheduled, adding peace of mind to your workday.

You can also put a digital lock on an interior door. This can keep children out of your medicine cabinet and give you the security of extra time if your home is broken into while you're asleep. Biometric locks are available for drawers, too, so you can selectively restrict access to prescription drugs, important papers, or other items you want to keep private. You can also use facial recognition to access these areas, just like unlocking your iPhone.

There is a wide range of price points and features on different systems, from DIY-friendly packages you can pick up at your neighborhood home center to more sophisticated systems available through a technology integrator or a national builder. As any professional will tell you, it's crucial to change the default password on any digital security device or system to a unique set of letters and numbers that no one else will be able to guess.

Higher-priced systems often come with technology that's harder to hack, as well as higher reliability and ease of use, and can be set up by a technology professional who knows how to keep intruders out of your home network and personal data. These may be worth considering for greater peace of mind if you have valuable artwork or sports gear or are living in an area more susceptible to break-ins.

There are potential drawbacks to digital security systems, particularly those that are mass-marketed. It isn't necessarily your own video doorbell that will create issues, although with some companies leveraging users' personal habits and data for revenue, it's impossible to predict how your comings and goings might be exploited for marketing purposes.

Some of these systems have also been shown to be vulnerable to hackers, which can in turn make you vulnerable to cyber or physical crimes. The major companies behind them create updates to foil intrusion when they learn about problems—often after victims have publicized their losses—so if you do feel the pros outweigh the cons of having off-the-shelf technology, be sure to keep your system and app updated.

ENVIRONMENTAL PROTECTION

Keeping criminals out of your home is one way to keep you safe. But it's also important to keep out other intruders, like unwanted water, smoke and fire, carbon monoxide, and radon. Building codes already mandate smoke alarms for your living space. In many areas, carbon monoxide detectors are also required. In too many tragedies, follow-up investigations found that alarms and detectors weren't working, often because the homes' occupants hadn't replaced batteries.

A smart home system can alert you to battery replacement needs before the alarm starts chirping. It can also alert you to a kitchen fire sooner if you're in a remote part of the house or yard, and to issues through your phone while you're at work or traveling.

Radon may be one danger you haven't heard of. Like carbon monoxide, it's undetectable without a sensor. It is a slower-acting gas that forms naturally in soil, rocks, and groundwater but is the second leading cause of lung cancer after cigarette smoke. Radon can enter your home through cracks and gaps in its walls and foundation. Basements are especially vulnerable. You can install a smart-home-controlled radon detector, which can alert you to issues whether you're home or away.

There are also smart home sensors for a broader range of indoor air quality hazards, including volatile organic compounds (VOCs) that result from home products like paint, furniture, carpets, and electronics off-gassing into your environment; particulate matter from fireplaces, cooking, and smoking; and even outdoor exhaust entering your home through open windows. Some of the more sophisticated systems tie in with smart home air filtration systems that will automatically activate when a pollutant is detected.

Another environmental risk comes from water intrusion. You might not realize there's a leak until water starts pouring through a wall or ceiling. By then you might have an unpleasant mold issue on your hands. If the leak built up unseen while you were away, you could find your home covered in it.

Mold isn't necessarily a health hazard to everyone (except when its spores contain mycotoxins), but it can be a problem for adults and children with respiratory issues or allergies to it. For everyone else, it's a disgusting cleanup chore.

New smart home systems that detect leaks and faucets left running are worth considering, especially the ones that shut off your home's water when they come across an issue. This is especially helpful for seasonal homes and unoccupied rentals.

LIGHTING

Lighting is tied into some smart home security systems, with various safety benefits. You can time them to turn on and off on your typical schedule while you're away, thus fooling a casual thief into thinking you're at home when you're actually surfing Australia, running the New York City Marathon, or summiting Denali. Security lighting can be triggered by an unauthorized attempted entry, spotlighting an intruder before he gets into your home. Lighting can also be linked to turn on when you arrive home, creating a safer entrance.

Voice control systems let you turn lights on and off with a command rather than fumbling for a switch in the dark, potentially avoiding a stumble. You can also create themes with voice commands, like

WELLNESS TIP
If a smart home system is not an option, changing your bedroom and bathroom light bulbs to warmer hues—now widely available at home centers—is an affordable alternative.

"Relax" to dim them, "Bedtime" to turn them off, "TV" to adjust to watching your favorite shows, and "Leave" to set them on automatic scheduling for while you're away.

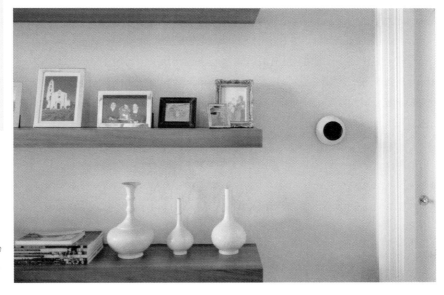

Smart home systems with voice control and privacy protection can help older adults live independently.

The latest, most wellness-focused advance to smart home lighting is called humancentric or circadian lighting. These refer to the level of color temperature, with brighter, bluer, cooler lights being better for daytime tasks like work and study, and softer, warmer light healthier past sunset. Too much blue light at night can overstimulate your brain and interrupt your sleep cycles, according to health experts.[1]

Since it's not practical to change light bulbs twice daily, tying your lighting into a smart home system that adjusts the color temperature automatically through the day can have definite benefits for your health and wellness.

CLIMATE CONTROL

Smart home thermostats are popular for saving energy and controlling your home's heating and cooling systems through your phone or tablet. They can also have wellness benefits, allowing you to lower the temperature to a healthy level while you're asleep, for example.

Some systems can be geofenced, meaning that the location setting in your phone will let the system know that you're approaching or departing from home. The advantage of this feature is that it can be set to warm your home before you arrive and turn the system off automatically when you leave.

Radiant floor systems, which are an option for heating your home or a room within it—bathrooms are especially popular—can also be smart-home enabled, so you can program your radiant floors to warm before your standard wake-up time, making for a happier encounter between your bare feet and bathroom tile.

Climate comfort isn't just about temperature, however. Humidity is a major factor in your health and comfort. Desert heat, or a home's own air-conditioning or heating system, can remove humidity from your space, causing skin, throat, and nasal issues. You can tie smart home–enabled humidifiers into your system to turn on and off automatically or by voice command.

Finally, your smart climate system can be tied in with your smart security system to protect your home's valuables, furniture, floors, and artwork against mold or excessive dryness. You can integrate your security system to automatically turn off your HVAC system should a door or window be left open so as to prevent mold-generating condensation, the drying out of a wood floor, or damage to an expensive work of art.

SMART HOME APPLIANCES

Smart home technology is making its way into appliances as well. Connected washers and dryers can let you know when your laundry is done or when you need to buy more detergent. Connected ovens can be preheated from your office, receive recipe instructions, and read bar codes on packaged foods. Connected ranges and cooktops can also communicate with connected range hoods to turn on to the right speed when you're cooking and let you know if a burner has been left on if you walk away.

Connected refrigerators let you peer inside via smartphone app while you're at the grocery store. So far, though, most product developers haven't been able to install cameras in the crisper drawers, so health-conscious shoppers won't know if they need more fish, fruit, or vegetables. They also haven't installed cameras in the freezer yet, so it's anyone's guess if your teen or spouse finished the last of the frozen bananas you were wanting to enjoy after a hot afternoon bike ride.

It's up to you to decide whether knowing there's only one yogurt left in the fridge or starting your dryer from the gym is worth the added cost of a smart appliance.

SMART HOME FIXTURES

There are now connected faucets with voice control, which is great for reducing germ spread in your kitchen and avoiding wasted water, but most are not yet able to accommodate requests for hot or cold. (This capability is starting to show up now.) Voice control technology has the potential to enhance wellness—especially in shared spaces like kitchens, powder rooms, and kids' bathrooms—when fully hands-free operation and temperature control are possible. It's also helpful to someone with arthritis or Parkinson's, which can make faucet operation difficult.

Another smart home fixture with wellness potential is the bathroom mirror, which can become a master suite hub for your smart home capabilities. You can operate blinds for privacy, regulate your thermostat for comfort, adjust your lighting for function, engage or disarm your security system, and connect to your phone for your favorite news or music.

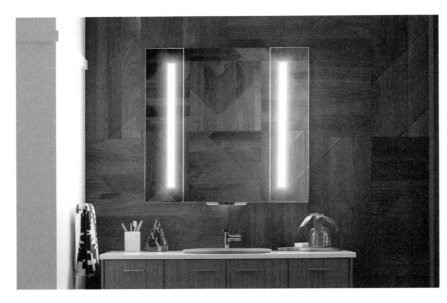

Smart bathroom mirrors are becoming hubs for news, entertainment, smart home systems, and personal wellness data.

Manufacturers and academic researchers are working on systems that can provide health information on your smart mirror as well, tying in with your scale and recording changes to keep you on track. Much of this technology is being tested and showcased at trade shows for industry input but is not yet commercially available. Stay tuned!

One connected bathroom fixture that is already available is the digital shower. You can program your favorite temperature and spray mode and start your shower from a button, app, or voice controller. Someone sharing the shower can preset his or her own modes. The shower can be started from your bedroom and paused when it reaches your settings, saving both time and water. Some shower systems on the market include waterproof Bluetooth speakers to play your favorite tunes, news, and weather and traffic reports, getting you ready for your day with greater efficiency.

SMART HOME AMENITIES

Smart home controls can help you create the home environment you want with a single command, operating your lighting, window coverings, and entertainment, security, and climate systems. Let's say you want to be able to turn on your favorite music, warm and dim the lights, turn on the fireplace, and close the shades when you walk in your living room after work. With many voice-controlled home automation systems, you can program all of those operations to happen when you program in a theme and then say a key word like "Relax." A programmed "Good night" sequence and verbal command tell your system to turn off the lights, activate the home's alarm system, adjust the room's temperature and humidity, and close the blackout shades. All of this is possible and available now.

Voice-controlled shades, alarm, security, and temperature controls are ideal for users with mobility issues. While you may associate smart home features with young adults, seniors find them extremely helpful in living independently. Sensors installed under the flooring and tied into smart home systems can alert a caregiver if someone has fallen at home or hasn't gotten up at their usual hour, so that no one has to remain immobilized or ill for hours or days without help.

Voice-enabled programming makes home automation easy to use for everyone from children to the elderly. Gone are the days of complicated remotes, touch screens, and four different buttons to operate your home. Now almost anyone, including the blind, can play music, close the shades, secure the house, and adjust the thermostat to their comfort level—without an engineering degree.

SMART HOME ISSUES

All of this technology comes at a price, including its purchase, installation, security, and maintenance costs. It also provides hackers possible access to your home and data, and potentially provides manufacturers and their business partners private information that you may not even realize is being shared or sold, as noted in the security section above. (This is typically an issue for off-the-shelf packages rather than professionally installed systems, which have different business models.) Privacy is a potential wellness issue, particularly as it relates to personal health and fitness information that can impact your future employment prospects and insurance costs if it becomes available to hiring managers.

Smart appliances and fixtures cost more than traditional products to purchase and require more expertise to install and repair. Some come with remote diagnosis capability from their manufacturers, somewhat addressing the repair issue. However, if a fixture or appliance has a one- or three-year warranty and you plan to keep it for ten or fifteen years, you're going to need a repair pro who can fix it later at your own expense. That might require more expensive, non-DIY-friendly expertise than you might think.

These are all issues to research before purchasing or installing smart home technology, and they definitely merit discussion on risk reduction with the technology professionals you hire. Privacy is a wellness feature, and losing it can be stressful and costly.

Be sure to discuss data privacy and network security when shopping for smart home technology.

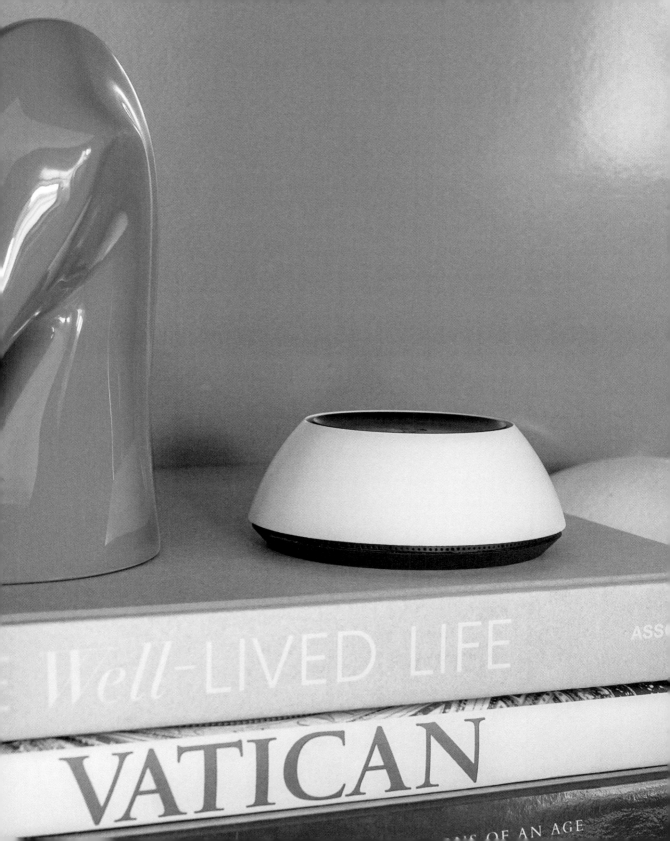

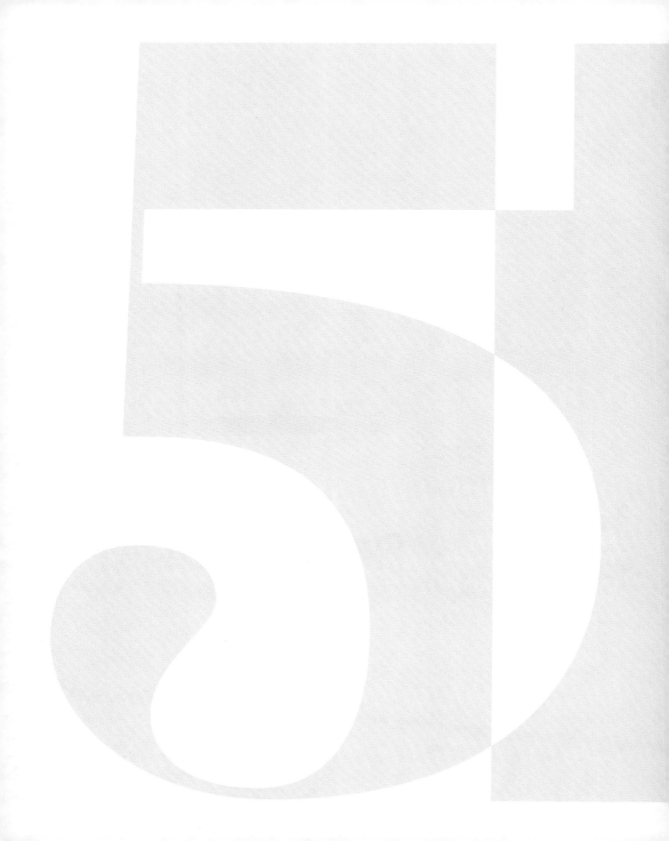

ENTRYWAYS

How do you feel when you walk up to your front door? Is your home's entrance welcoming? Does coming home after a workday or vacation make you smile? Ideally, the answers are great, yes, and yes. Your home is your sanctuary, and entering it should bring pride and delight. Both benefit your emotional health.

FRONT ENTRIES

Approaching your front door should also be a safe, easy experience for you, other household members, guests, delivery people, and mail carriers. That means the paths from the curb and driveway (if applicable) are free of trip hazards like broken pavers or uneven concrete, and well lit for nighttime arrivals and departures. It also means that your entrances and pathways are well maintained to avoid hazards like fire ants and are clear of pet waste, thorns from nearby hedges, and scooters or bicycles.

Your address should be easily visible from the curb, even at night. This might mean letters on the curb that can be seen in a car's headlights or illuminated numbers on your home's wall. Either makes

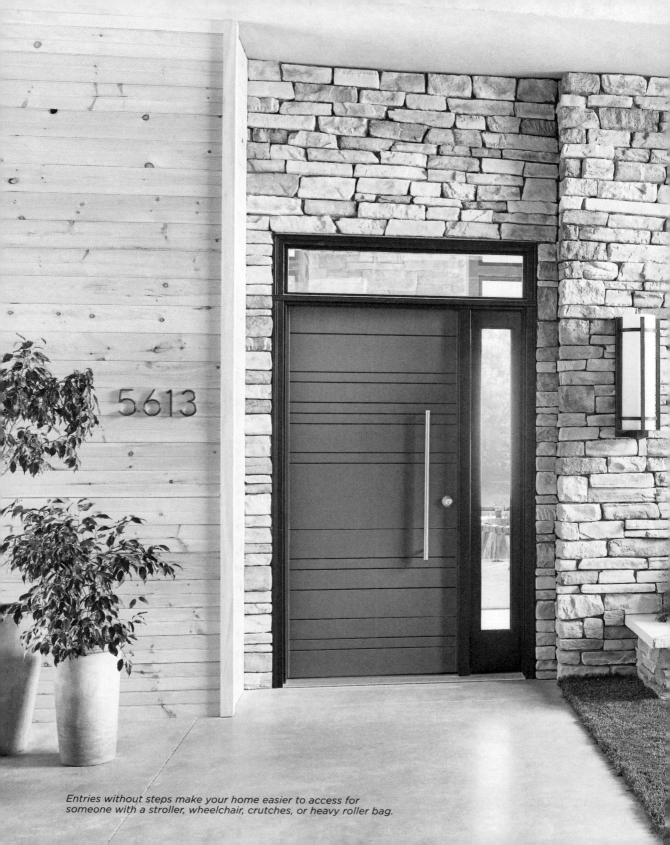

Entries without steps make your home easier to access for someone with a stroller, wheelchair, crutches, or heavy roller bag.

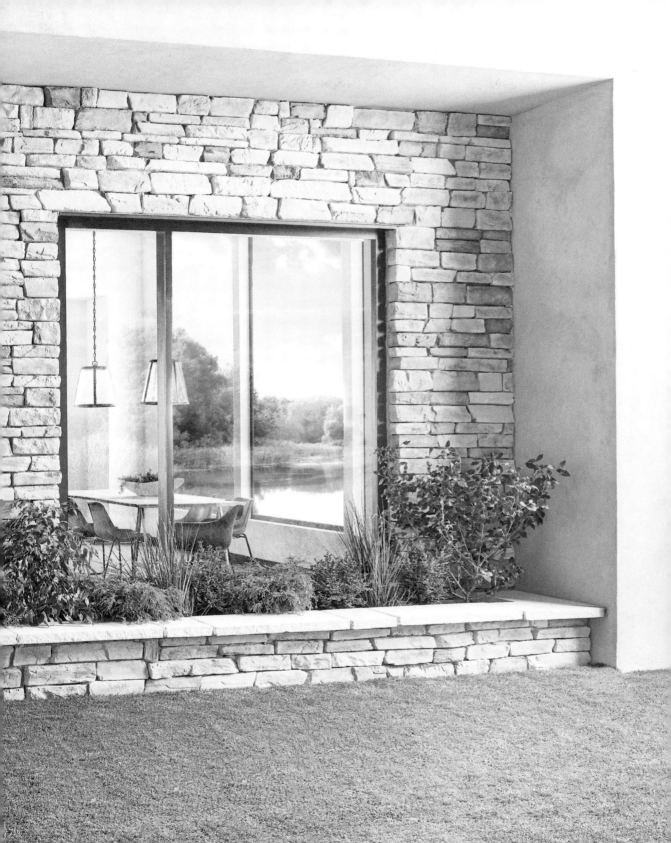

it possible for guests, food delivery or ride share drivers, and, most important, first responders to find your home quickly.

If you have stairs leading to a landing, porch, or deck and your front door, you should also have a stair railing, ideally on both sides, and the steps should be built to code, kept in good repair, and clear of toys, snow, ice, and debris.

HOUSE CALL

Seniors who fall are at risk for brain injuries, hematomas (large bruises due to internal bleeding), fractured leg, foot, or pelvic bones and fractures to their wrists or forearms by trying to break their fall. On an emotional level, seniors often experience an increased—and sometimes debilitating—fear of falling after an incident occurs, regardless of whether they were injured. This can seriously impact their peace of mind and quality of life.
—*Brittany Ferri, MS, OTR/L, CLT, CCTP, registered occupational therapist, Rochester, New York; simplicityofhealth.com*

If possible, it's ideal to have an alternate entrance without stairs or other barriers to getting into your home for someone with a wheelchair. That may not be you or anyone in your household right now, but making your home "visitable" by guests with mobility challenges is a plus for you and them (and potentially increases your home's resale value). It could also be very helpful if you or someone else in your household has an injury or illness that makes it harder to use stairs. An entrance without steps is considered barrier-free and is also convenient for parents with strollers and for anyone with heavy, wheeled luggage.

If you have space close to your front door, it's ideal to place a small bench there. This can serve multiple purposes. First, it lets you or someone else in your household put down packages to reach for keys. Juggling bags or boxes while trying to get a door open can be awkward. Second, it provides a guest with a place to sit while waiting for you to come home. Third, for anyone with fatigue, a bench offers a spot to rest for a moment.

Some entryways are larger, with seating and side tables. These are often associated with traditional homes and porches and are wonderful additions to any residence! They give you a place to relax outdoors, converse with neighbors, and spend time at home with family and friends. (Read more about these in chapter 6, "Outdoor Living Spaces.")

GARAGE ENTRIES

You may use your garage entry more frequently than your front door. That's especially common in suburban homes where people drive most places. You'll want to make sure that you can move easily between your car and your home's garage entry door if you've added storage along the side walls or have two vehicles. That's also pretty typical these days. Some homeowners have so much stuff in their garage that they can't park their cars inside. (See chapter 18, "Garage," for garage ideas.)

The last thing you want to do when coming home is trip on something between your car and your house or knock something heavy off a shelf onto your foot. Plan at least three clear feet between any storage you're adding to the sidewalls of your garage and where your vehicle needs to be parked for a safe walkway. That applies to both your driver's and passengers' sides. You may live alone and have just one vehicle, but there's always the delightful prospect of guests and their cars.

ENTRY MATS

Every entry door to your home should have its own mat for scraping muck off your shoes before walking inside. This can be an opportunity to personalize your entrance with color, pattern, or even wit. There is no shortage of choices, from inspirational to humorous. Whichever you choose, though, the mat should be heavy enough not to slip or blow away, durable for years of use, low-maintenance for hosing off when needed, and well suited to your climate.

Entry mats at a home's front door can be a curb appeal enhancer, both for your delight and that of your visitors. Don't underestimate the ability of a simple, single element to make you smile! And don't underestimate the ability of a delighted smile to lift your spirits.

Entry mats at a back door or garage entry can do the same for you and your household, perhaps with some sly, private family humor unsuited for the more public-facing front door. Whatever welcomes you home and shifts your mood from work to relaxation and the pleasure of your space works.

INTERIOR ENTRIES

Once you're inside your home, you have another entry, perhaps one from your garage and another at your front door. It—or they—may be large or small but should also be welcoming and free of trip hazards. Choose the entrance you use most often to hold jackets and coats, umbrellas, pet needs, and shoes.

You should create this as a highly functional space that makes leaving quick and easy and coming home pleasant and convenient. Some homes have room for storage benches or "locker" walls, with space for each household member to put their gear. That's ideal if you have the room and budget. If you don't, hooks for each person's coats and bags can work, and a shared bench for backpacks, briefcases, and sitting while removing shoes can meet the need.

Why remove your shoes at the door if you don't do this habitually now? you may be wondering. There are several good reasons. First, you're not going to track in dirt, bacteria, toxins, and pebbles from outside. Second, you'll cut down on cleaning time. Third, you'll save your floors from scratches and other damage. The habit of removing your shoes when you enter your home also creates a mental shift from outside world to indoor sanctuary.

An organized entry with shoe storage keeps your home cleaner and calmer.

You'll want a place to store those shoes out of the walk path so you can put them on quickly to head outside. That can be a floor tray with a lip all the way around if you're in a snowy climate, an easy-to-clean moisture-tolerant mat, or a piece of storage furniture.

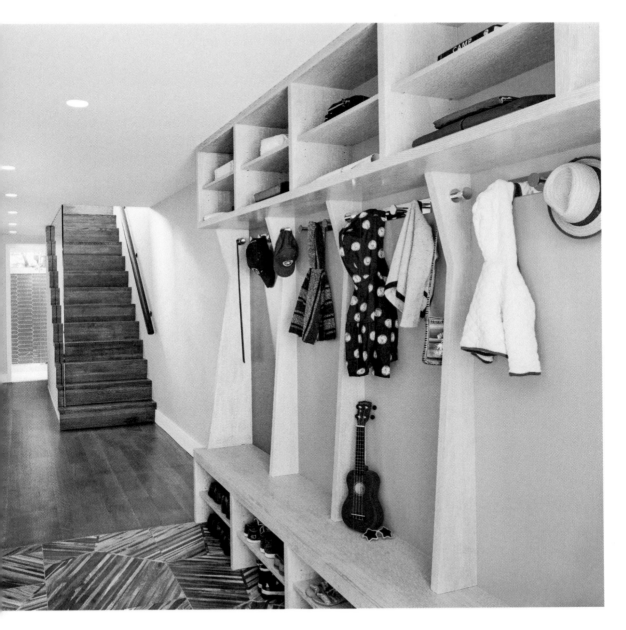

Shoe benches are ideal if you have the room, as they provide both a place to sit while you take shoes off and put them on and a place to hold them off the floor. Just make sure the one you choose has room for the type of shoes you wear regularly. For some folks, that's boots, which may not fit into standard cubbies. Thick-soled running shoes may not, either.

You need to ensure that you have thirty-six inches of room to walk past the shoe bench, tray, or mat to access stairs, adjacent rooms, and your home's entry doors. It's great to be able to store slippers for yourself, other household members, and guests in the same shoe space, so you can easily change footwear from outdoors to indoors. This is particularly true in cold or rainy seasons when your socks are likelier to get wet.

ENTRYWAY GEAR MANAGEMENT

If you participate in the kind of sports where your clothing, shoes, and socks get wet or muddy on a regular basis, removing and cleaning them outside—possibly in your garage if you have one—before entering your home is ideal.

If don't have a garage or exterior hose, you can add a machine-washable mat and portable bin to your entry area that can be carried into your laundry area to avoid tracking messes through the rest of your home.

These mess catchers can be as stylish as the rest of your residence. You want the first area that greets you when you return home to be attractive as well as functional. Storage furniture should complement furniture or cabinetry in the adjacent rooms. If the entry leads to your kitchen and the cabinets are white Shaker, for example, it's nice to have white or Shaker styling on a shoe bench or locker wall. You don't need to go matchy-matchy, but coordinating finishes and details will give your home a more pulled-together look.

You can also create a pulled-together look by continuing the flooring from the adjacent rooms into the entryway. As long as it's durable and low-maintenance, it should work in that area too. This makes your overall space seem larger than if you selected a separate material for the entry.

It's likely that a back entry connecting a garage with a laundry area or mudroom will be in a utilitarian tile, and a front entry connecting with the home's living spaces will be a more decorative material like wood. You can make any of them work, although grout will present more of a maintenance challenge, and wood or laminate can be damaged if not protected from outside elements. That's another reason to remove your shoes when you come into your home.

Another element to add to your entry to protect it from the elements is an umbrella holder. If there's space in the garage, and that's the entrance you use most often, it can be simple but attractive. If your household and guests regularly enter through your front door, an attractive umbrella holder that has enough space and a style that coordinates with the rest of the space should be selected.

Your entryways may be designed just for quick passage. That doesn't mean they have to be drab. Since they are the first places to welcome you home, take the opportunity to add art that you'll enjoy looking at every time you come in. It could be something personal, like a photograph of yourself at your last race or on vacation, or a piece you bought from a local artist and had framed for your indoor entries. It could be a medal rack or trophy shelf for your garage entry. Every time you enter your home, your mood should be lifted.

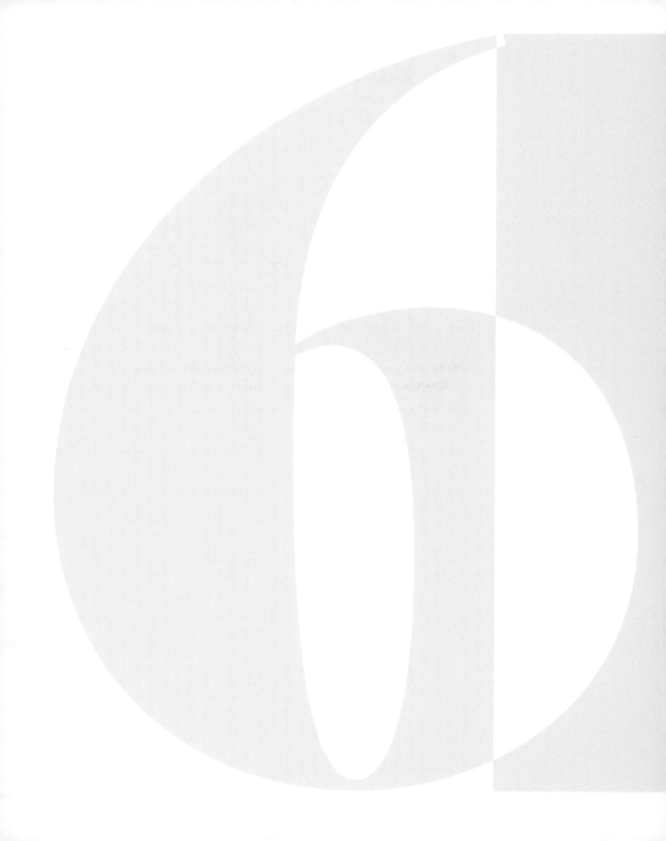

Outdoor LIVING SPACES

I f your home has its own outdoor living space, you're fortunate. You can use this area for relaxation, gardening, meditation, exercise, socializing, and stargazing. Even a small balcony affords an outdoor break. Natural light can improve your concentration, mood, stress levels, vitamin D intake, and possibly even healing, according to some research,[1] so take the opportunity to go outside—if just for five minutes at a time!

Even if you don't have your own outdoor space, you can enjoy shared community areas for these benefits—without ever having to push a mower or fix a sprinkler head. (There are some benefits to not having a yard!) Taking a quick break from chores or work-at-home tasks to bathe yourself in sunshine and enjoy a burst of nature can be restorative. There's wisdom in the common advice to stop and smell the roses.

Some property management companies and neighborhood associations are facilitating the creation of community gardens where residents can have their own plots for fruit, vegetables, flowers, herbs, or whatever will grow in those conditions. It's worth asking about starting a community garden if there isn't one in your complex.

If your building doesn't have grassy areas that can be repurposed for planting, ask management whether the roof can be used for an outdoor garden and seating areas. These will enhance its value and appeal to other prospective tenants, so the answer may be yes.

If you have your own space, these ideas can help you create a wellness living area at home. Your starting point is analyzing the space's location, sun exposure, potential uses, security, and privacy. A fenced yard presents different opportunities from a front porch. Let's take a look at each space and how you can make the most of it for your health and wellness.

HOUSE CALL

Spending time in nature—even for brief walks—has many benefits. These include lowering cortisol levels (a hormone that becomes elevated under stress, and causes more rapid aging); strengthening the immune system; lowering blood pressure; enhancing memory function; diminishing anxiety; and building a sense of well-being. When combined with other practices that can be performed at the same time (such as meditation while walking, or mental journaling what one is grateful for), one's time in nature becomes a particularly powerful way to mentally reset and recharge.
—Forrest Talley, PhD, psychologist, Folsom, California; forresttalley.com

FRONT PORCHES

This is part of your home's entryway and should offer safe passage and curb appeal, as mentioned before. Depending on its size, your porch may also offer room for a settee, chairs or porch swing, and side table. These are great features for creating a welcoming space where you can socialize with family and neighbors. A porch this size is almost certainly going to be covered, creating the opportunity for adding ceiling fans—and possibly even misters for very hot climates—to cool seating areas. The porch may also be screened for keeping out insects.

Given their openness to the street, front porches are generally used for social activities rather than exercise. That doesn't mean you can't take a moment there for a quiet gratitude meditation on the joys of your life and community, and there are definitely wellness opportunities in spending time with friends.

If you're building a home or adding or remodeling a porch, you'll be faced with a decision on what to clad it in. Choices generally sort out to wood or wood alternatives. Wood may be pine or redwood, two popular options. Redwood costs more but doesn't need to be treated for insects or weather; pine does. Cedar is another weather- and pest-resistant wood, but it is also expensive. Both will save you time in the long run, as you will not have to spend your evenings or weekends repairing or resealing them.

Bamboo is a wood-like decking alternative made from grasses, not trees, that comes in different grades, from composite and strand versions that are both blends of bamboo and man-made materials to solid bamboo planking. Solid and high-quality composite are generally the most durable, but some need to be sealed to keep their glues from breaking down with time and sunlight.

Many homeowners choose low-maintenance and durable materials that look like wood but can be vinyl or composites made from recycled plastic and wood scraps. These will vary in quality. If you're installing the porch yourself, you'll need to familiarize yourself with local codes governing safe disposal of faux wood sawdust. You may want to use a specialty mask as well, so you're not breathing the chemicals emitted by those materials while working with them. Their off-gassing is less hazardous outdoors, where it can dissipate into the open air, but you don't want to be inhaling these fumes during the installation process.

DECKS AND PATIOS

Your deck or patio may offer more privacy, being on the back or side of your house, and may also provide an overhead structure for hanging outdoor draperies. These can add both privacy and some protection from the sun.

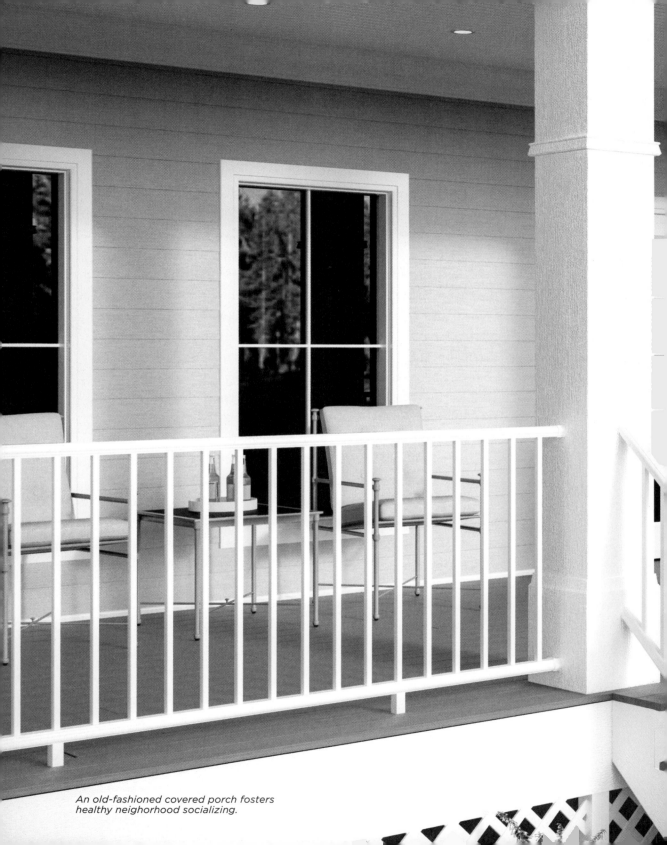

*An old-fashioned covered porch fosters
healthy neighorhood socializing.*

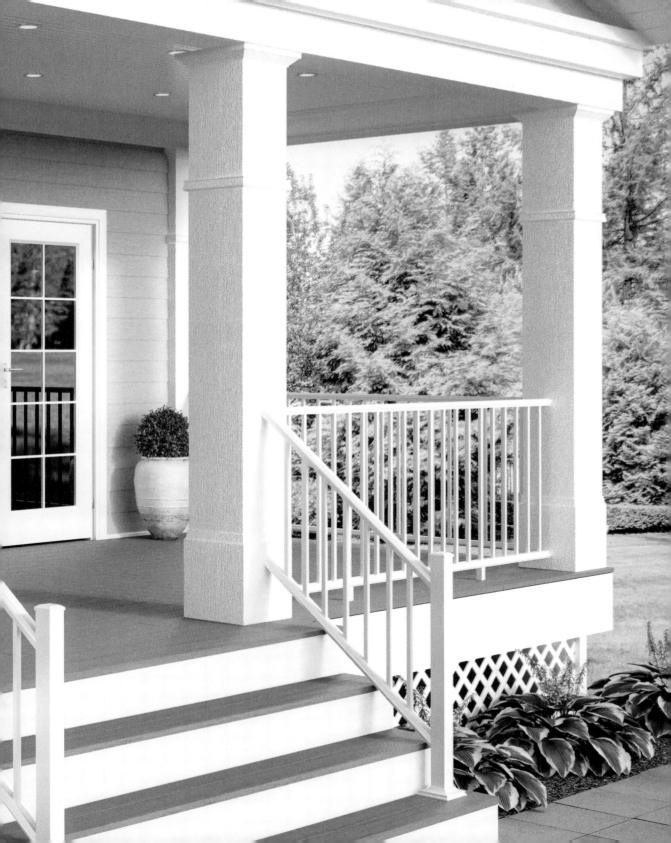

That can create a safe outdoor space not just for socializing but also for yoga, meditation, exercise, or napping.

You'll have the same choices for cladding your deck if you're building or remodeling one, although it may be fully or partially uncovered. (That means more maintenance if you're opting for wood, and you will need to factor in slip resistance.)

Some patios are merely extensions of the home's slab foundation and made from the same concrete. You may be able to cover yours in an outdoor-rated floor tile if it won't create a transition issue with the entry threshold from indoors. If you want a decorative look without tile, you can have the concrete professionally painted or stained.

Rooftop decks often use raised pedestal pavers that allow for quick drainage and removal, if needed, to get at roof issues. They are typically made of cast concrete, although porcelain pavers are getting popular. They are stronger, lighter, and decorative.

You can cover an outdoor floor with outdoor rugs. These are durable and moisture- and fade-resistant. If they get soiled, your outdoor rugs can generally be hosed off. They can personalize your space while protecting bare feet from being scorched by hot surfaces under a burning sun. Larger decks and patios may use outdoor rugs to create separate lounging and dining areas.

People who grew up in the country may miss their fields of green. Artificial turf can't truly replace those, and there are some health warnings associated with artificial turf, including its components and maintenance materials, but the new versions can provide a soft, maintenance-free section of grass in a small outdoor living space. No, it won't attract honeybees or butterflies, and you won't have that delicious scent of fresh cuttings, but you won't have to spend your weekends mowing it, and it can help allergy sufferers spend more time outdoors.

If your deck or patio isn't covered, you're going to want to look for sun protection to really be able to enjoy it during the hotter months. This can be a freestanding umbrella or an awning attached to your home.

The former is a better solution for anyone renting, as you'll be able to take it with you when you move. If you are considering an awning for a home you own, it's worth looking at one that can be remote-controlled to shade an area in advance of your backyard party, or one that comes with meters that retract automatically when the wind picks up. That can protect your investment in windy seasons and regions.

Another option for sun protection is an outdoor canopy or gazebo. These can also offer some privacy and protection from insects, depending on how their sides are constructed. You'll need to determine whether it can stand safely and securely on your property and not violate any homeowner association rules. If they're allowed in your neighborhood, consider anchoring your freestanding structure so unexpected high winds won't turn it into a dangerous flying wing.

YARDS

Your home may have an open or fenced space beyond your deck or patio. Depending on how much space there is available, and how level, you may be able to set up outdoor games like badminton or volleyball, enjoy a round of catch with your kids, or play fetch with your dog. These can all be great fun and good workouts but can expose you and your companions to ticks, mosquitoes, bees, and wasps. Ticks and mosquitoes carry diseases, and stings can create health issues for those with allergies.

Keep your grass mowed and clear of leaves to minimize tick contact, and empty any standing water, even small amounts, to keep mosquitoes from breeding in your yard. If you have a bee or wasp nest, you can steer yourself and visitors clear or have it professionally removed.

BALCONIES

These are often small spaces that just give residents a chance to step outside. If you have room for seating or dining, look for outdoor-rated furniture that will comfortably fit with room to walk around them. Consider that balconies don't usually offer full privacy, so that might limit your activities. You can still enjoy this space as an escape from indoors—especially with sunrise or sunset views, birds chirping, or a fountain gurgling, and gentle breezes cooling an afternoon read—as your own outdoor café where you can sip an iced drink with friends, or as an alfresco meditation corner. It's probably not going to be your strapless tanning space, though!

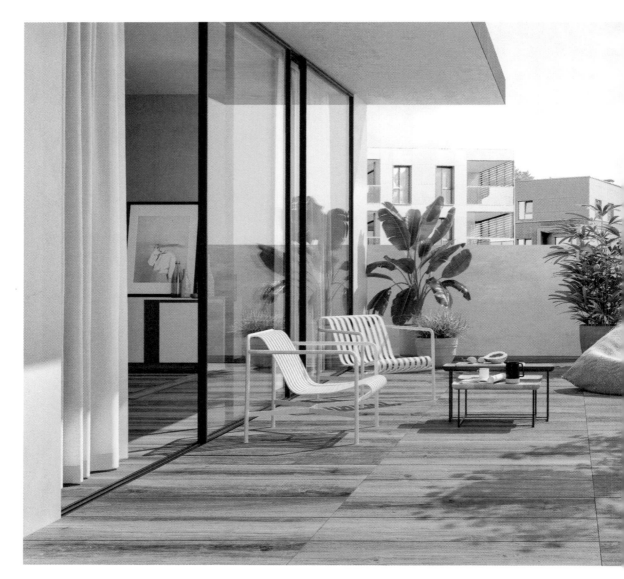

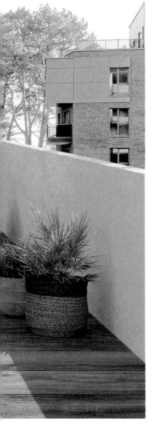

If you have wall space, you can add outdoor-tolerant artwork to personalize your balcony. If your balcony doesn't overlook nature, you can add some with potted plants or a green wall. An outdoor rug can also enhance the space.

POOLS AND SPAS

Pools can be great for cooling off on hot summer days and for teaching your children how to swim. They can add beauty, a fitness option, and outdoor enjoyment to your home. They can also add danger. Hundreds of children drown each year in pools. Laws and common sense say to fence yours in and have a door alarm leading to the pool area.

If you're buying or renting an older home, make sure the drain is properly covered so that no one gets trapped by it. This has been law since 2007, but it never hurts to make sure it was followed before risking your life or anyone else's in your pool.

If you're adding a pool to your home, you may be offered a choice of traditional chlorine or salt water. Saltwater pools still use chlorine, but much less. (They also have much less salt than the ocean.) Saltwater pools may have some wellness benefits for people with allergies or asthma, health experts say.[2] And if you find chlorine irritating, a saltwater pool may be a good option for you. It may cost more to install but can save you money on maintenance.

Your pool may not be long or straight enough for lap swimming, but water aerobics can give you a good workout. You can also do water walking or running, which athletic coaches sometimes recommend for people recuperating from injuries to keep up their cardio levels without the pounding of pavement.

Balconies can be enhanced with comfortable seating areas and plants for quick, healthy "nature breaks."

Your spa can be a great relaxation and recovery spot, providing you have no health conditions, such as pregnancy, that may make the use of a spa inadvisable. The heat and jets can soothe sore muscles after an intense workout, increase circulation, reduce arthritis and fibromyalgia pain, lower stress levels, and improve sleep.

Though tempting, it's not really a safe idea to enjoy alcohol in a hot tub or spa. In addition to the potential for broken glass from a dropped bottle or wine goblet, you can also make yourself dizzy or dehydrated. If an adult beverage is an absolute must, drink it from a shatterproof glass, step out of the water to let your body cool off every fifteen minutes or so, and invite a companion for safety. That has its own social wellness potential.

Given the dangers of drowning, your spa—like your pool—should be secured from children when you're not there to watch them. You'll also want to keep your spa regularly and properly maintained so that it doesn't become a bacterial hazard.

POOL BATHS AND OUTDOOR SHOWERS

If you're buying or building a home with a pool—or one near the beach—you'll find having an outdoor shower or pool bath useful. Outdoor showers are just what they seem: they're a space to wash ocean or pool water off your body so you don't track and drip it into your home. They're often simple affairs, with just controls, a showerhead, and maybe a soap dish and divider or curtain for a little privacy.

Pool baths are more elaborate, as they also provide a sink and toilet. What distinguishes them from traditional secondary bathrooms is their direct access from the pool area of your home. This enables pool party guests to rush in and out without tracking water through your home. It's a convenience for them and a little less hosting stress for you. If your family loves using your pool, consider adding a hook for each person's towel to hang on between uses and wash day.

OUTDOOR FURNITURE

Even covered spaces can get hot in summer months, so consider that metal furniture can be uncomfortable to touch. If you're considering a metal set, be sure to include back as well as seat cushions. Wood, wicker, and rattan are attractive alternatives, but all of these natural materials need maintenance, something you may not want to spend your free time doing.

Resin is a low-maintenance outdoor furniture alternative. It can be made to look like wicker or wood, doesn't emit toxins, and won't fade or chip. Poorly made resin furniture can crack or split, though, creating a safety issue.

Many styles of outdoor furniture call for cushions. Fortunately, there's a large selection of outdoor-rated upholstery that will stand up to moisture, sunshine, sunblock, and spills. These are great options for easy outdoor living.

OUTDOOR KITCHENS

Grilling food has been popular since humans first discovered fire, and is still a mostly healthful way to cook. There is a wide range of grill types available, with different types of cooking features and using different types of fuel. What you cook will certainly enhance the health quotient of your meal, but research shows that grilling high-protein meats and fish over open flames can, in certain circumstances, allow cancer-causing smoke to permeate your food.[3] You can reduce this hazard by avoiding fatty flare-ups with a water bottle, cooking longer over a lower temperature, and lining the grill with perforated tinfoil. Marinating meat or fish before grilling also reduces this risk. Grilling fruit and vegetables instead avoids it altogether.

In addition to grills, there are now also pizza ovens, outdoor food warmers, and outdoor-rated wine refrigerators to ramp up your outdoor dining experience. If you're creating a built-in outdoor kitchen—especially one with a ceiling—it's definitely worth considering a ventilation hood to redirect cooking smoke up and away from people so that family and guests don't get covered in it while you're cooking.

Outdoor pizza ovens have gotten very popular in recent years. Just as with grills, there are portable or built-in models, from affordable to luxurious, with many using wood as fuel for traditional "wood-fired" appeal. What you make your pizza crust from and top it with will have the biggest impact on how much salt, sugar, and fat your meal has, but your homemade pizza has the potential to be a healthful home-cooked meal, and pizza parties can make for great socializing.

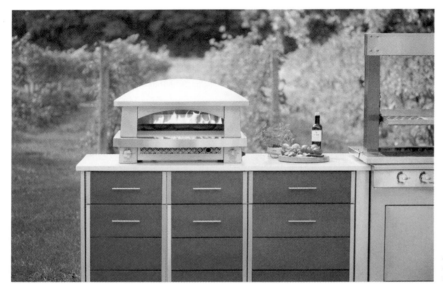

Wood-fired pizza ovens and low-maintenance cabinetry make healthy outdoor socializing easier.

OUTDOOR PLANTS

Outdoor plants can be beautiful, fragrant, and delicious, depending on what will grow in your area. You don't need a garden to grow plants outside, either. Containers will work for many varieties, and self-watering containers make success easier. Greens like lettuce and spinach will grow in pots. Tomatoes, cucumbers, carrots, and beans will too. That sounds like a salad in the making!

You'll want to choose vegetables that prefer the light level your outdoor space offers and compatible water levels to grow in a shared

WELLNESS TIP
If you already have trees or another nature feature available, consider placing a comfortable seating area nearby with shade or a view for relaxation.

pot. A horticulturalist or garden center expert can advise you in this regard. You can grow figs, apples, peaches, cherries, and other fruit in containers as well. These can be enjoyed on their own as healthy snacks or mixed into home-cooked recipes.

Roses, gardenias, lavender, peonies, and freesia in pots can all add scent and color to your space. Rosemary, mint, and sage also add fragrance to your space and flavor to your cooking. These can all be grown in containers if you don't have a garden. Once again, check with a plant pro on which will work well in your light and shade levels.

If you have a deck, patio, or balcony to grow plants on, you can add beauty and wellness to your space. If you have room to plant an actual garden, or access to a community garden, and you enjoy gardening as a healthful hobby, your wellness potential is even greater.

As noted earlier, some homeowners and property managers are creating green walls in their outdoor spaces. These living vertical gardens can improve air quality, enhance your feeling of wellness, act as sound barriers, and absorb heat. If your green wall includes herbs and greens, it can also enhance your cooking. Siting a green wall near your indoor and outdoor kitchens makes meal prep more convenient and flavorful.

If you have the room and opportunity to plant trees in your yard, you will reap more benefits than just the shade they will eventually provide. Trees improve air quality, cool the air around them, and reduce stress. They also attract songbirds and can create privacy around your home's perimeter. When it comes to trees, your soil, climate, and exposure matter tremendously. It's also important to understand the trees you plant and their root systems so that they can be strategically placed where future growth won't cause issues with your home's foundations, concrete flatwork, retaining walls, and other structures. A professional arborist can advise you on what trees will grow where you live and where to place them.

KITCHEN

Kitchens are often called the heart or the hub of the home. Real estate agents consider them a home's most important selling tool. You should think of your kitchen as your home's fueling station. Its most important function is enabling meal preparation. And preparing and consuming healthful meals are among the most important factors in your overall health and wellness. Food fuels your brain and basic bodily functions. It also fuels your workouts and provides the nutrients you need for overall performance in life. If you're lacking nutrients, you'll find yourself fatigued more easily, less able to focus, and less able to perform whatever task you're attempting.

You may also pay your bills, manage your household, and entertain guests in your kitchen, but prioritize its fueling functions above all. What does that mean exactly? It means that your kitchen should be well equipped, well lit, and well organized so you can safely and easily create healthful meals there.

PRIORITIZING MEAL PREPARATION

Making meals should be easy and convenient in your kitchen, because the essentials you need are close at hand, quickly located, and easily reached. If you have to hunt for the utensils, spices, or the perfect pot for the job each time you want to cook your favorite foods, you'll find yourself wasting time and feeling frustrated.

Too many busy people skip cooking because it feels like a hassle—and when kitchens are cluttered and poorly planned, it is. But this doesn't have to be the case, and shouldn't be. Eating food you prepare yourself helps you control your calories, sodium, sugar, fat, and portions—all of the essentials of successful fueling—much more easily than dining out or ordering restaurant meal delivery.

Optimizing your kitchen as a winning space for meal prep will also optimize your health, training, and fitness. There are changes both large and small that can make a big difference—whether you rent or own—and these will help you enjoy using this space much more.

ZONING YOUR LAYOUT

How your kitchen is laid out can have a tremendous impact on its efficiency. If you're not remodeling, either because the time isn't right for such a large project or because you're renting, you're not going to move walls, change appliances, or add built-in accessories to the cabinets. However, that doesn't mean you can't improve the room's layout. You can start by reimagining the space.

Think of your kitchen in terms of zones. You have a food storage zone, which includes your refrigerator and pantry space. You have a cooking zone, which includes a range or cooktop and ovens, ventilation hood or over-the-range microwave with built-in vent fan (also called a micro-hood), and possibly a warming drawer. Last but not least is your cleanup zone, including your sink, your garbage disposal, your dishwasher, and possibly a trash compactor. Your cleanup zone is also part of your prep space, as it's where you'll clean fruits and vegetables, perhaps trim beef or chicken, drain pasta, and do other cleaning-oriented meal prep tasks. It's also where your trash will be stored between trips to the dumpster or curb.

These essential zones make up what used to be considered the kitchen's work triangle (before kitchens started expanding with islands and other features). Sometimes these zones are well planned by the builder, with the pantry and refrigerator close to each other for faster grocery unloading, and ample cabinet space near your range or cooktop for both pots and utensils. The dishwasher is always going to be next to the sink, as it shares its plumbing components, but it's ideal when there's also room for cutting boards in this zone and counter space for chopping and dish draining. This is also a convenient space for storing your dishes, glasses, and silverware, since it helps you unload the dishwasher with fewer steps.

What if your kitchen isn't well laid out, as is too often the case? By reorganizing the storage and counter space near its appliances and fixtures, you can make your kitchen work better for your needs.

MAXIMIZING YOUR ZONES

The first step is decluttering. The easy part is finding spaces outside the kitchen work zones for the piles of mail, bills, catalogs, kids' homework, and other paperwork that seem to grow effortlessly on your countertops. These stacks can create an eyesore that makes your kitchen less appealing to work in, taking up the counter space you need for healthful meal prep, making your counters less hygienic and more time-consuming to clean, and possibly becoming a fire hazard. Relegate them to a different area, perhaps by creating a "family landing zone" near, but not in, the kitchen. (That might be a family room cabinet with shelves for everyone, or cubbies for each family member in the household's daily entry hall.) You'll find your kitchen is much nicer and feels larger and more welcoming when its surfaces have been decluttered.

On to the next step . . .

Take a look at your small countertop appliances. Are you using them regularly? Are they helping you create healthful meals? If the answer is no to either question, consider moving these items to an out-of-the-way spot in your kitchen, like the cabinet above the refrigerator or microhood, elsewhere in your home, or to a donation center. If you use them sometimes but not daily or weekly, a pantry shelf can be dedicated to holding them. At the end of this reorganization process, your countertops will be decluttered and you will have much more space for meal prep. Your kitchen will also be a much more pleasant space to use.

It's time to look at your cooking tools. Go through your cabinets and pull out utensils and pots and pans that you're no longer using. If they're in good condition, they can be donated to charity. If they're damaged—especially if they're chipped, peeling nonstick cookware—they should be tossed.

Special-use cookware, like the paella pan, the turkey roaster, or the fondue pot that you only use once or twice a year, can be stored with the less-used countertop appliances in an out-of-the-way spot in your kitchen or elsewhere in your home. You may find you have much more cabinet space than you thought you did, and it's more useful than you had previously believed.

Now comes the trickier part. You're going to reorganize the cabinets you have so that the items you need are in the right zone. Let's take spices as an example. If you season food as you cook it, you're going to want to store your spices in your cooking zone, close to the cooktop or ovens. If, on the other hand, you do all of your seasoning right after you chop and dice, before you add heat, you may want to have your spices in your food storage zone with your other ingredients, or in your prep zone where you mix your ingredients.

Other storage is more zone-specific, like keeping your pots and pans close to the cooktop or range, baking dishes and trays near the oven, and cooking utensils closest to the appliance you'll be using them with most often. In an ideal kitchen, there are drawers next to those appliances to hold utensils and deep space for pots, pans, and other cooking vessels. Too often, though, kitchens aren't ideally planned. This can be overcome by repurposing storage with zoned organizers.

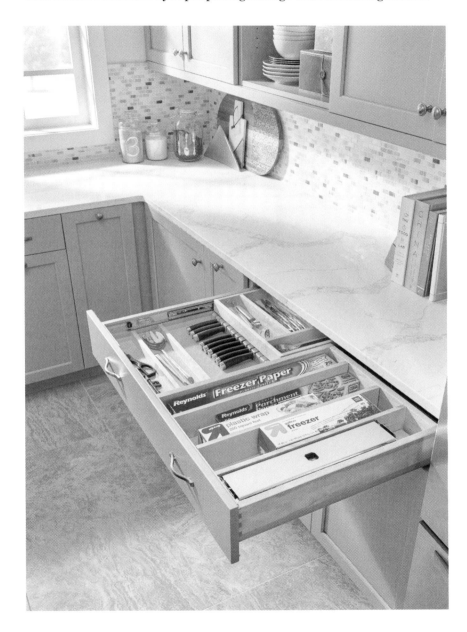

Maximize your kitchen with organizers that improve your storage and efficiency.

ZONE ENHANCEMENTS

If the builder failed to include enough drawers, you can add their equivalent with deep roll-out trays near the top of your base cabinets. If you're renting your space, add an organizer bin for utensils and potholders to the top shelf of your cabinet that can be easily moved onto the counter for convenience when you need its items. (One European cabinet manufacturer just showcased this concept with removable drawers.)

If you have a base cabinet near your stove with shelves that are too narrow for your pots and pans, you can reorient it with a side-mount pot and pan-organizing pullout. If that narrow cabinet is close to your sink and dishwasher, add a pull-out tray divider for holding your color-coded dishwasher-safe cutting board set. Renters can add a freestanding divider that doesn't need to be secured to the cabinet.

One of the most common kitchen complaints is lack of usable storage space, especially those useless "blind" corner cabinets where you can only see one side. A swing-out accessory can make the back of a corner cabinet just as useful as the front: no more kneepads and flashlights needed for finding what you forgot you placed there when you moved in!

Swing-out accessories and roll-out trays are especially beneficial for anyone with back issues, as they make base storage much more accessible. If you have older kitchen cabinets that still have their original half-depth center shelves, you can significantly increase your storage capacity by replacing these underperformers with full-depth roll-out trays.

Roll-out trays or pull-out units are also ideal for cabinetry-style pantries, as they let you see what you have much more easily than standard shelves. (That's how you avoid having umpteen cans of diced tomatoes dating back to the last millennium.) If you're renting your place, baskets or bins on shelves organized by food types will make a pantry cabinet easier to use, as well. These can also better organize a walk-in pantry that is either part of a rental or not able to accommodate roll-outs.

Roll-outs are beneficial for trash storage too. Trash cans will typically go into the kitchen's cleanup zone, and include a bin for garbage, with one behind it for kitchen recycling items like bottles and cans. The benefits of roll-out trash storage are that it can be closed off from toddlers and pets and won't get knocked over. There are models that have filtered lids if odor is an issue; these also work well in a nursery for diapers.

You can add storage to a small kitchen with organizers that install or hang on the back of a cabinet door. These can hold cleaning supplies under the sink or spices in a wall cabinet near the cooktop. Add them with an eye toward zone placement so that you're saving yourself steps when preparing your meals.

Backsplash organizers are another way to add storage and convenience to a kitchen you own. You can hang large utensils near your stovetop, for example, especially those like ladles that don't always fit well into builder-grade drawers. Backsplashes can also be used for getting paper towel holders, knife blocks, and other small items off your countertops. There are over-the-door holders for the former and in-drawer organizers for the latter if you're renting.

Ceiling space can be used for pot racks in especially small kitchens, or for those who like to keep all of their cookware immediately visible. That's an entirely personal choice. The trick is to know what works for you and plan accordingly, so that all of your kitchen space is optimized for easy, convenient, pleasant meal preparation.

SPECIALIZED ZONES

You can also designate specialized zones, depending on your cooking and nutrition preferences. For example, let's say that juicing is one of your passions. You can create a juicing zone where you'll store, wash, and prep the produce you juice, along with holding your blender, juicer, and accessories. Depending on the layout of your kitchen, this can be close to the sink or refrigerator or on an island.

If you're creating a juice zone as part of a kitchen remodel or new construction project, you can plan an area with counter space for preparation, a prep sink for rinsing produce, a compost bin for scraps, a fridge drawer for produce requiring refrigeration, roll-out bins or shelves for nonrefrigerated items, and an appliance lift for a heavy juicer and blender. This creates a self-contained, superefficient prep space for your healthy juicing habit.

You can create baking zones, canning zones, and healthy snack zones for your kids with the same space-planning approach to grouping prep areas and storage organizers around fixtures and appliances to most conveniently meet that need.

If you take supplements or medicine that should be consumed with food, you can designate a supplement storage zone in your kitchen so that your prescriptions and vitamins are always handy when you're ready to eat, and so that drugs that need to be refrigerated are close by in a cold space.

Where you keep your supplements and medication in the kitchen will depend on where you have room to install an organizer; you want to set it up so that you can easily read each label and perhaps organize your supplements by time of day so that you can always quickly grab what you need on schedule.

CABINETRY AND FURNITURE

If you're planning on remodeling your kitchen, you'll probably be choosing new cabinets, and possibly some freestanding furniture items. While you'll primarily be considering style, durability, and price—all important details—it's good to consider what they're made of and how they're finished. Style is just one factor.

Will your cabinets require just a quick wipe after cooking or will they need endless fingerprint (or pet nose print) removal? Is the trendy gloss worth the extra time spent keeping it pristine? For those who love traditionally styled kitchens, is that elaborate door style going to require cotton swabs to dust or degrease? Is it worth the time you could be spending in nature rather than indoors cleaning?

When it comes to furniture, beware of inexpensive online imports! It's not uncommon for them to off-gas tremendously, especially in their first weeks in your home, and the low quality may not make them safe, durable additions to your household.

You may also be looking at upholstery for banquettes or stools. This is not the spot for delicate, dry-clean-only fabrics! You want these materials to be durable and low-maintenance.

If you're working with a designer or upholsterer, you can request nontoxic, easy-wearing furniture, fabrics, and other products. If you're choosing on your own, you can use an online database search for certified nontoxic materials. (See the Checklists and Resources section at the back of the book for more information on accessing updated website links.) It could be worth the extra investment to get pieces that are better constructed and will be healthier in your home.

For those who enjoy relaxing or socializing in their kitchen, a couch is a nice addition. It can be a space for enjoying a cup of green tea or coffee while choosing recipes to make over the weekend, for enjoying a restorative nap, catching up on your book club selection, or for spending time with a treasured friend. Choose an easy-to-care for, durable fabric that only has to be wiped clean if food or drink is spilled on it. If you're going to use it in place of a bench at your table, customize it with higher legs to bring you to a comfortable dining height.

COUNTERTOPS AND BACKSPLASHES

Countertops are hard-used surfaces and are sometimes hard to maintain as well. Old-style four-inch-tile countertops have lots of grout to keep clean. Granite and marble countertops need to be kept sealed. Wood countertops also need regular special care. If you have those in your kitchen, you'll need to maintain them properly for appearance, durability, and food safety.

If you're planning a kitchen remodel, you may want to look for durable materials with lower maintenance requirements; after all, this is precious time you can be out running, hiking, cycling, or just forest bathing rather than resealing your kitchen countertops!

One of the most popular materials for kitchen tops is engineered stone, also known as quartz. As noted in chapter 3, "Material Choices," it will never need to be sealed and is highly heat-, scratch-, and stain-resistant. This is a very family-friendly surface. Orange or tomato juice spills are not going to hurt quartz tops. Neither is the hot pot your teenager sets down occasionally without a trivet.

Another up-and-coming material for kitchen tops is porcelain slab, also called sintered stone. They're made from material similar to the old tile countertops you couldn't wait to get rid of but without their drawbacks. The lack of grout means no tough cleanup jobs. The porcelain material means a hot pot or knife scratch won't hurt it. Porcelain can also extend into an outdoor kitchen, which most engineered quartz can't.

Both quartz and porcelain can be good options for a low-maintenance, wellness-focused kitchen. Another wellness option to consider is solid surface, one of the few repairable countertop materials; this can be a real benefit to households with active kids. Like quartz and porcelain, it's nonporous and never needs to be sealed, but it is going to scratch more easily. (Some scratches can be buffed out by a nonprofessional.) It is also not rated for outdoor kitchens.

Backsplashes have become popular spots for personal expression. That's great for emotional wellness; there's nothing like walking into your space and seeing a beautiful tile mural that speaks to your passions, travels, or memories. It adds to your pleasure in using your kitchen. At the same time, some design concepts can create more challenging cleanup work—e.g., lots of white grout behind a cook-top—and that should be factored into your planning process. Perhaps place that creative accent where it won't be splashed by miso soup or tomato sauce.

An alternative idea is to run a low-maintenance countertop surface up the wall or opt for scrubbable paint as a more budget-friendly option. You can add cheerful personality with playful paint colors like sunny yellow or energetic orange, and change it back to neutral if you're renting and decide to move. Choose a high-quality, scrubbable no-VOC paint that will clean easily and won't off-gas into your kitchen to preserve your home's air quality.

FLOORING

The other major surface in your kitchen is its flooring. In many modern homes, the same material extends from the kitchen into the living spaces. That makes it a larger investment to change. If you are going to replace what you have, here are some ideas.

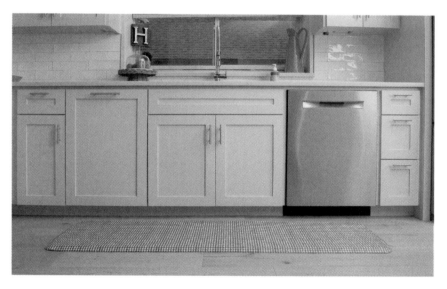

An anti-fatigue mat can make long meal-prep sessions less wearing on your joints.

Porcelain is a popular option for its durability. When installed with minimal grout lines, maintenance is also minimized. When selecting tile for kitchen floors, you want slip resistance to reduce the chance of a painful fall. The only disadvantage of tile in a space where you may spend hours standing at the counter or stove preparing meals is its hardness. After a while, you're likely to feel pressure from that hardness in your back, hips, knees, calves, and feet. The last thing you want to experience is unnecessary wear and tear on your body when taking care of your nutritional needs.

Wood is another popular option for kitchen flooring. If you choose it, you might find a distressed finish less stressful to live with, especially with an active household and large pets. Cork and linoleum are other good kitchen options, and softer underfoot than wood or tile.

LIGHTING

Kitchens need two kinds of lighting: ambient and task. Ambient light is provided by sunlight streaming through windows or skylights and overhead lights for darker kitchens and general night use. These light sources will illuminate your space overall but are not usually enough for close work like reading recipes, measuring ingredients, and using knives. Those require task lighting.

Islands, peninsulas, and breakfast bars are often lit by decorative pendants. Sometimes, though, the builder just put in a recessed light that doesn't provide enough illumination for your needs. It isn't very difficult to replace one of these with a pendant to bring the light closer to the work surface. If you choose an LED model, you can potentially also increase the amount of light where you do your meal prep without increasing your energy load. You can even do this in a rental if you don't mind switching back to the can lights when you move out.

Another good source of task lighting is under-cabinet lighting. These are typically LEDs that are mounted beneath wall cabinets. With a trend toward open shelves in place of cabinets, you can look for LEDs that attach to shelf bottoms instead or come built into the shelf. These shine light directly onto your work area, which recessed ceiling lights don't do nearly as well.

For those not in a position to install this lighting permanently (and have it on its own switch), there are battery-operated LEDs and plug-in models. Whichever mode works best for your needs, this is a worthwhile add-on to a well-used kitchen—and may make the difference between perfectly julienned vegetables and jabbed fingertips.

APPLIANCES

Appliances are the brains and muscle of a kitchen. At the most basic level, they'll preserve and cook your food, keep your kitchen grease- and odor-free, and clean your dishes. If you're renting an apartment, these are the basics you can expect. Perhaps the oven has a convection setting to keep food from drying out and cooking it faster. That's a plus.

Cooking

If you're choosing an oven for a new home kitchen or remodeling project, it's worth considering a convection steam oven, also called

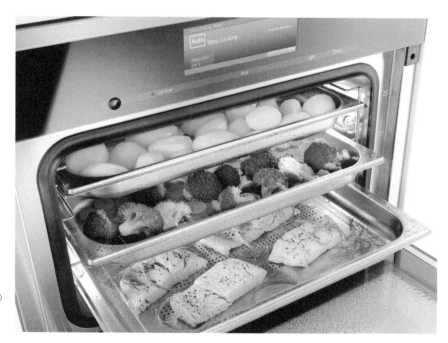

Convection steam (also called combi steam) ovens are ideal for healthier cooking and reheating.

a combi steam oven. Steaming food does an excellent job of preserving its moisture and nutrients. Adding the convection feature means adding the browning, roasting, and baking features you want. This is a powerful appliance that can improve the quality and taste of your cooking, but will cost more than a standard oven. If you don't have the room or budget for a built-in combi steam oven (or you're renting), you can find a countertop model that will work for smaller dishes or households. If that's not feasible, a steamer basket offers a simple solution.

HOUSE CALL

Different cooking styles can help retain or deplete the nutritional value of food. Steaming is great because it helps to preserve food's micronutrients. Other methods, such as boiling, can leach water-soluble vitamins. While there are many different cooking styles that can provide a variety of flavor outcomes for your food, steaming is a great way to ensure that the nutritional quality remains intact.
—Martha Lawder, MS, RDN, registered dietitian, Sacramento, California

When it comes to cooking surfaces, many traditional cooks request gas. Induction is an alternative worth considering for wellness-conscious, serious cooks. It is much faster than even high-BTU gas burners, saving you time in meal preparation. It won't heat up your kitchen in the summer, making cooking more pleasant in the hotter months. And since only the surface directly under the pot or pan heats up, there's less chance of a child accidentally burning a hand. Fire risk is also dramatically reduced, as clothing and kitchen towels won't start burning if they touch an induction cooktop. (This is a huge benefit if your kitchen has an over-the-range microwave oven, as so many do.)

After cooking your food faster, induction will be much faster to clean up as well. Food does not bake onto it as it can with gas and electric burners, making it a snap to maintain. Finally, if your kitchen is small, its smooth surface can double as extra counter space when not in use.

Induction cooking is available on cooktops and ranges; it can even be built into some porcelain slab countertops for a sleek, edgeless cooking area. There is one caveat for induction cooking: If you have a pacemaker, check with your doctor about whether the electromagnetic fields of an induction cooktop will interfere with it. In most cases, you'll be fine, but do ask first as a safety precaution!

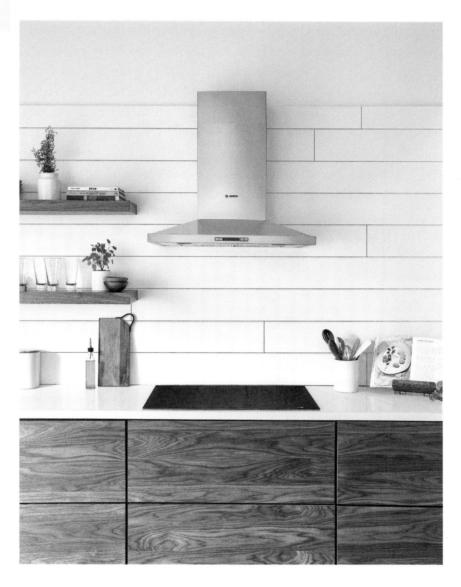

Induction cooking is a high-performance, family-friendly technology.

Cooktops paired with wall ovens tend to be more ergonomic than ranges—a big help for wheelchair users, anyone with chronic back issues, or those with less upper body strength—but require more room, which your kitchen may not have.

If it does, you can install an oven at a height that's easier for you to use and more comfortable than the close-to-floor oven built into a range. Some wall ovens have side-opening French doors that can be especially helpful for wheelchair users; they won't have a heavy oven door landing in the chef's lap or making access to the interior a longer, harder reach.

A warming drawer, or the warming setting on a range or oven, will keep food warm and ready to be served for family members on different schedules, like kids at sports practice or a spouse at after-work yoga class or boot camp.

One cooking zone appliance that sometimes gets short shrift is the vent hood. Cooking ventilation is absolutely essential for pulling steam, odors, and grease out of your kitchen, thus improving its indoor air quality. Unfortunately, too many models are loud, inefficient, and hard to maintain. That makes them less usable and unpleasant to operate.

In recent years, vent hoods started getting combined with over-the-range microwave ovens. These microhoods tend to be especially noisy and often meet just the minimum ventilation requirements. They can also lead to uncomfortably hot handles or fire risks if your shirt gets too close to a gas burner while you're reaching into it. If you're stuck with one of these while you're renting or waiting to be able to remodel, at least use the vent fan— you do not want to cook without one! A quietly running ventilation hood or insert that has an easy-to-clean filter—perhaps even dishwasher-friendly—and vents outdoors will be your best option.

Downdraft vents tend to be less efficient than overhead models, although new technology is being introduced in Europe that promises superior performance with low maintenance when it eventually comes to our shores. Recirculating models are also less efficient than venting outdoors. Both are better than no ventilation at all, but an overhead hood is generally going to work best right now, and one that works with less noise will protect your hearing and make kitchen conversation easier.

Refrigeration

Apart from door configurations and finishes, refrigerators haven't changed dramatically over the decades. They have gotten more sophisticated in styling and offer some specialized storage bins and dispensing features along the way. What has changed most notably is the ability to customize your food preservation.

Built-in refrigerator columns let you choose how much fresh versus frozen food you want to keep in your kitchen, something that can be beneficial if you keep more of one than the other on hand than is typical, or if you need to keep certain foods separate for religious reasons. Customizing also lets you add under-counter refrigeration where it will be most helpful.

For example, if you prepare salads daily, you can add a refrigerator drawer just for fresh produce to an island installation for convenient meal prep. If you have children, you can add a mini-fridge with healthy drinks and snacks for them near where they do homework, so they don't have to go into the main fridge after school while you're cooking.

Cleanup

Dishwashers have made cleanup significantly easier in the decades since they've been introduced. Opt for the quietest model you can find, as it will make using your kitchen more pleasant while it's running. If you're a wine drinker, a china setting will be gentler on your glasses. If you have a newborn, a sanitize setting can be beneficial. If you use sports bottles (or baby bottles), bottle wash jets can be a nice feature.

If you have lower back issues or use a wheelchair, a drawer

dishwasher can be helpful. (Some accessible kitchens have raised dish-washers, but they don't work well except when installed on the end of a cabinet run.)

Newer models and detergents also mean that rinsing your dishes and cookware before loading them into the dishwasher is largely un-necessary now. This can be a huge time and water saver. Wouldn't you rather be spending that time relaxing after dinner?

Appliance Extras

A wine refrigerator with two or three zones will keep your bottles at the proper temperatures. Wine can be relaxing after a stressful day for those who can enjoy it without issues—and, according to medical research, moderate consumption of red wine can also have some real health benefits.[1] If you're a wine enthusiast without room or resources for a wine refrigerator, a wine rack in your kitchen can meet basic needs. (Just don't put it in an area that gets warm!)

A built-in coffee maker is another appliance worth considering for a kitchen remodel by those who take their beans seriously. Cof-fee does have wellness benefits, health experts say,[2] and some run-ners swear by it for prerace consumption. Being able to have a cup of espresso, cappuccino, or standard brew on demand—perhaps even with a programmable timer—certainly has its appeal. This is definitely a luxury appliance for someone craving the sleekest of kitchens. A good countertop model with the features you're seeking is a more than viable alternative.

If you are planning on adding a coffee maker to your kitchen, whether countertop or built-in, it's worth considering a water filtra-tion system for the best taste. (Your coffee will only be as good as the water you add to your beans.)

Countertop Appliances

In addition to portable induction burners and coffee makers, there are some additional small appliances that can enhance your healthful eating. One is a digital food scale. This helps with regulating your portion sizes and completing recipes. Look for a model that lets you zero out your container.

Another useful countertop appliance is a blender or food processor. There are specialized versions that do everything from mixing smoothies to making soup. Choose the features that make the most sense for how you cook and eat, but having even a basic model can help you prepare healthful food and drinks at home.

If you're renting, or not planning to remodel anytime soon, but you want the benefits of convenient convection and steam cooking, you can find a countertop oven enabled with one or both of these premium cooking methods.

Another countertop appliance worth considering if you don't have a built-in or outdoor version is an indoor electric grill. Former heavyweight boxing champion George Foreman popularized these in the last two decades, and now there are numerous models to choose from. Fruit and vegetables grill beautifully on these small appliances and are a healthier option than grilled meat or fish. Look for a model with dishwasher-safe plates for time-saving convenience.

Two more appliance types definitely worth considering are the slow cooker (often known by one of its most popular brand names, Crock-Pot), and the multicooker (most often known by the brand name Instant Pot). Slow cooking lets you prepare healthful meals without added fats and without having to tend to the food while cooking. Using the low heat setting will tenderize meats and keep them from drying out, soften vegetables, and maintain nutrients within the food. Multicookers add steaming, rice cooking, and other healthy modes like sous vide, depending on the brand and model you select. Many busy home chefs appreciate its speed as a cooking powerhouse on busy weeknights as well as its slow-cooking options.

Whether you opt for a slow cooker or a multicooker, be sure to choose a model with an automatic keep-warm setting. This will switch the appliance from cooking to warming when the food is fully cooked, so you can have dinner ready to eat when you come home from work. Many busy home cooks love the convenience of prepping their ingredients, turning the appliance on before leaving the house and coming back to the aroma of a seasonal stew or vegan jambalaya.

Here are a few safety issues to consider when using a slow cooker or multicooker: (1) Make sure it's sitting on a level, clutter-free surface, like a countertop. (2) Don't refrigerate the ingredients in the insert; use a separate container. (3) Don't use the appliance with an extension cord or plug that's frayed or damaged in any way. (4) Keep it out of the reach of pets and children while it's cooking.

For those who can't give up the occasional fried food, an air fryer lets you cook with minimal oil, reducing fat and calories. While air fryers beat deep fryers, grilling, steaming, and roasting are healthier cooking options overall. An air fryer may be one of those less used small appliances you move to a higher cabinet or shelf, rather than keeping it on the countertop where it can stare at you.

SINKS AND FAUCETS

Sinks are among the most essential of your kitchen features. They are used to wash produce and bathe infants, drain pasta and clean hands. They're often employed to scrub pots and pans that won't fit in the dishwasher. How well they perform depends on their size, shape, and material.

If you're redoing your kitchen, you want a model that will work well and clean up easily. That can be a 16- or 18-gauge stainless steel, granite composite, solid surface, quartz, or ceramic sink. Each of these will resist scratches and give you years of use. An integral sink—built into the countertop—is often the easiest to clean after use, as there's no crevice or lip for food to get caught on. These can be made of porcelain (in porcelain slab countertops), quartz, or solid surface materials. If an integral sink isn't an option, an undermount sink is the next easiest to maintain. This can include farmhouse (also called apron-front) sinks.

Some new sink models include accessories that sit on ledges, making meal prep, entertaining, and cleanup easier. These are called pro sinks, workstation sinks, or chef sinks. Having the accessories ready to use is a plus when you're in a hurry or handling complex tasks. Chef sinks come in sizes ranging from compact single-bowl models for small kitchens to massive multi-bowl workstation models for the larger kitchen and more serious home chef (and budget). Given the growing popularity of these sophisticated sinks, there's increasing availability and affordability. Just be sure to choose a material that will hold up under hard use.

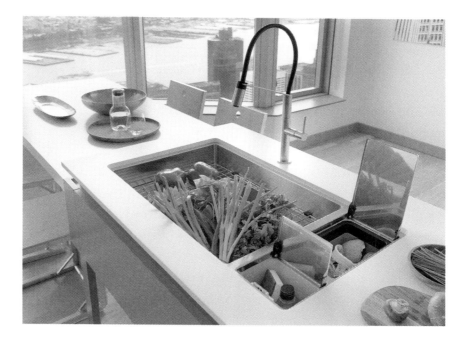

A pro-style chef sink makes meal prep and cleanup chores faster and easier.

Kitchen faucets are another essential that have added performance features. Multi-spray modes and pullouts are common now, making prep and cleanup more convenient. Hands-free operation is becoming more popular and has some wellness benefits. The less surface contact, the fewer germs that are shared between household members—a huge benefit in cold and flu season—and the fewer foodborne bacteria that are left behind during the cooking process.

Hands-free faucets are also easier to turn on and off when you're holding a heavy pot or pan. You can often activate them with an elbow when your hands are occupied. The newest models have voice activation. This is the greatest convenience of all, as you can turn on a faucet as you approach the sink, even telling it how much water you need; but as anyone who has struggled with being understood by a voice assistant can tell you, there's still work to be done on these technologies.

One consideration to think about when choosing a faucet is its finish, especially if it's not a hands-free model. One that offers spot resistance will be easier to keep clean, especially in a household with children.

It's also worth considering a second faucet for a multiuser workstation so two cooks can prep or clean up at the same time. Space them at an interval that will work for both of you so that no one is getting bumped while handwashing paring knives!

PLANTS

Kitchen plant life has moved off of the windowsill and into special placement within the work zones themselves. There are wall-based cabinetry systems designed to help plants grow with built-in drainage and lights. Those are generally intended for the herbs and greens that you'll use in cooking. There are even built-in appliances with climate control for growing herbs and microgreens. There are also less elaborate island and wall systems that can accommodate live plants for the same purpose. All of these options add healthy elements to your kitchen with the welcoming benefits of plants—as well as their nutrients for fresh meals.

WELLNESS TIP
There are now countertop appliances and packages like AeroGarden, Ivation, and Hamama that will grow plants for cooking in your kitchen when you rent or aren't ready to remodel.

KITCHEN SAFETY

Half of all home fires start in the kitchen, often during the dinner hour, and often involving the cooktop or range. Surprisingly, electric ranges have a higher incidence of cooking fires than gas ranges. (Perhaps the presence of an open flame spurs more caution around them.) The leading cause of home cooking fires is unattended appliances, which means that too many people are putting something on a burner, turning it on, and leaving the area. Don't!

Vent hoods can be fire hazards as well, especially if they weren't properly installed, sized, or vented outdoors. Most commonly, they can create fires when grease builds up inside the hood or the vent. If you're not sure how to maintain the model in your kitchen, look for its manual online or contact the manufacturer.

It's helpful to have a class B fire extinguisher close to the kitchen for use on a very small stovetop fire, and know how to use it. However, if a fire is fast growing, get yourself and any other occupants out of the home quickly and call your local fire department.

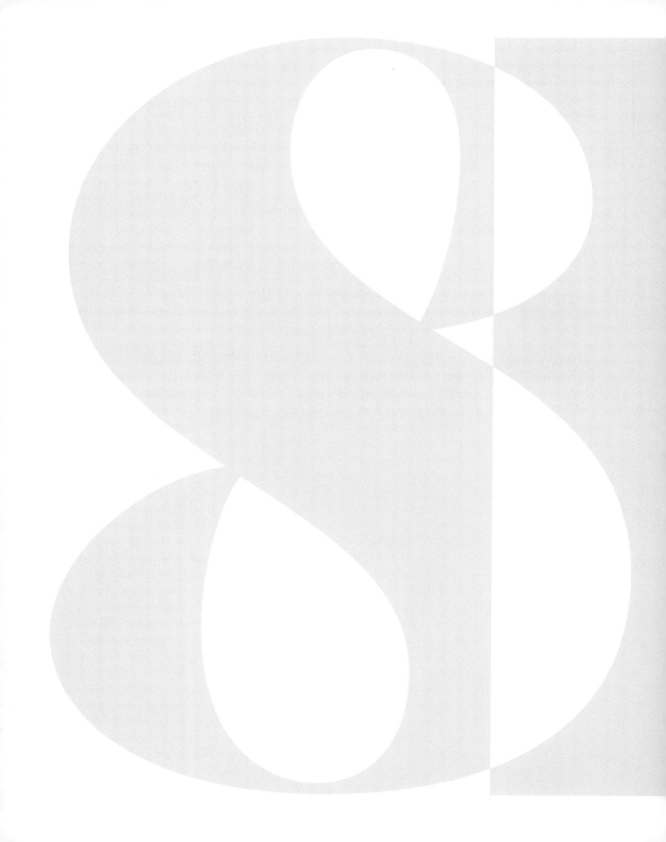

HOME OFFICE/WORKSPACES

The ranks of telecommuters keep growing, from people working full-time at home to people who may work one day at home and then four at the office or on the road. Does either describe your job?

Perhaps you do work outside the home but use a home office space to pursue a degree or certification, write a blog or novel, or run a small business or e-commerce site for extra income. Is your workplace down the hall from your bedroom? Or does it comprise a desk and chair in the corner of that bedroom? For many, their workspace is wherever they can find a corner to concentrate. There's no single right spot, but there are real considerations in making it a healthy one.

The more hours you spend working from home in whatever capacity, the greater the need for it to support your physical and emotional well-being. But how? The basics of just about every home office space—whether dedicated or shared with other uses—include seating, work surface, lighting, storage, and technology. The extras are soothing surroundings, easy access to nature, and opportunities for creative expression.

Considering how many hours some of us spend working, it's

important that our workspaces be ergonomic. What does that mean? It means that the furniture or equipment works with your body to help you achieve necessary tasks. If you've ever experienced neck pain or lower back pain at the end of a workday, there's an excellent chance your workspace is not ergonomic. If you work from home, you can change that.

WORK SURFACES

Your at-home work surface may be your kitchen counter or dining room table, but standard dining chairs and counter stools are not necessarily ideal for long hours of work. In fact, sitting for hours isn't

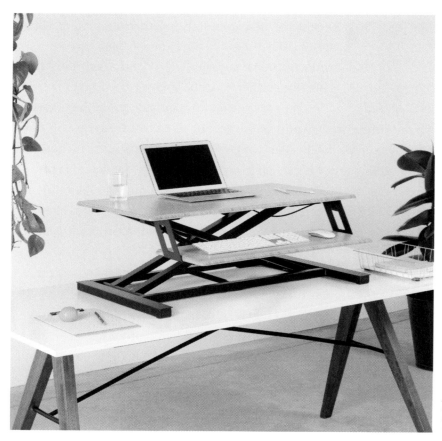

A desk riser makes office work more ergonomic and healthy with sit/stand flexibility.

WELLNESS TIP
Adjustable risers
let you change the
height of your work
surface through
the day so you can
alternate sitting
and standing.

ideal, either, as many health professionals are realizing.[1] Let's look at some ideas and alternatives.

Stands and risers can elevate your keyboard to a comfortable standing height, and sit on a desk, counter, or table. Monitor arms can adjust your screen to an ergonomic height and secure to any of those surfaces as well. These options all come in numerous styles and sizes, even accommodating dual screens if you need those for your tasks. It's also helpful if you share your workspace with another user whose height is different from yours—or if you have children of different heights who do their homework at the same desk.

There isn't one material that works better than others for work surfaces. Something that looks good and cleans easily, like wood, solid surface, or laminate, is usually a good bet, especially during cold and flu season, when you'll be doing more wiping than usual.

Your work surface's size will be determined by the nature of your work. One benefit of a wider desk, if there's room, is the potential for more legroom below so your knees aren't banging against legs, side panels, or file drawers all day. You want to be able to roll close enough so that your screens are in a comfortable field of view and you can reach your supplies without stretching uncomfortably.

Ergonomics experts have mixed thoughts on the benefits of wrist rests.[2] The consensus is that if they keep your wrists from bending during extensive keyboard work, and rest under your palms or the heel of your hands, not your wrists, they can be beneficial in reducing fatigue and repetitive stress.

HOME OFFICE SEATING

If you're spending hours every day in a chair, it needs to be comfortable and supportive. Adjustability is hugely beneficial in achieving ergonomics. That means a backrest, armrests, seat height, and lumbar support that can be moved into position to accommodate your body's dimensions.

Health professionals recommend adjusting the seat height so that your thighs are parallel to the floor and your feet rest flat on a footrest or the floor.[3] Your armrests should be at a height that keeps your shoulders relaxed.

Some recommend a balance ball with stability ring (so it doesn't roll away from you), or a balance stool (which can work well at a kitchen counter, too, as it will easily tuck underneath when not in use). Balancing activates your core and improves your seating posture. That can reduce spine impingement from sitting for hours in a traditional chair. If a balance ball isn't appealing, a balance disk on your existing chair is another option.

Standing and moving when you can during your office time are also ideal. These can be achieved by raising your work surface and computer, or getting a wireless headset that lets you pace and stretch your legs during phone calls. They can also be achieved by using a treadmill desk, although it's not a full-time option for everyone. It's much easier to talk on the phone while walking than it is to create architectural plans, for example.

Sometimes just standing and moving at regular intervals during your workday are all you need. They require only enough floor space to stretch, pace, march in place, or turn up the music and "dance between drafts" of whatever project you're working on. (You're home: no one's watching!)

If you stand for long periods while working, especially on a very hard floor like tile or concrete, it's worth considering an anti-fatigue mat to stand on so you can ease the stress on your body. You'll see these in stores for cashiers.

An ergonomic desk chair, sit-to-stand desk, task lighting, and plants add wellness potential to a home office.

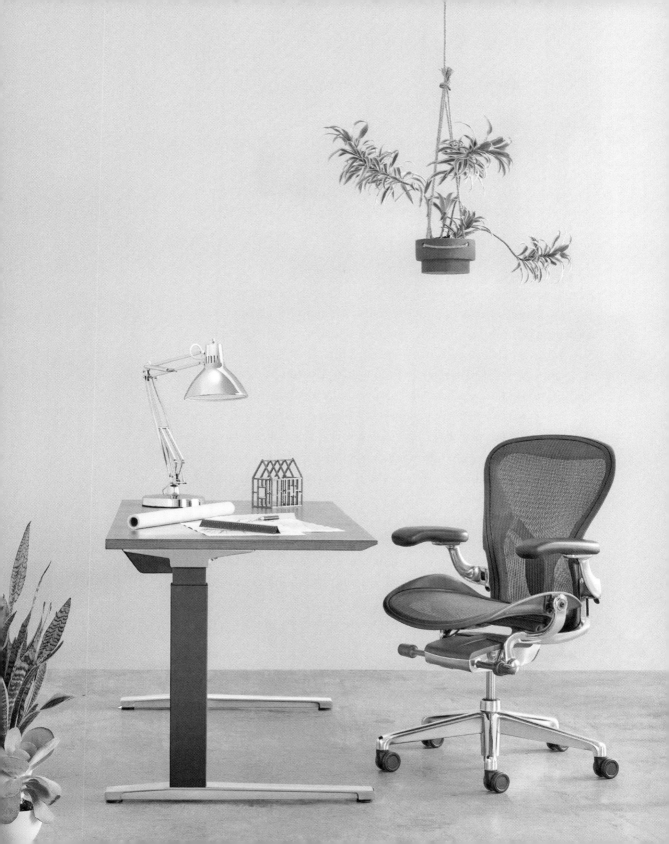

STORAGE

Even if you've managed to go completely paperless in your work life, you're still going to need space for your basic supplies, computer, and possibly a printer-scanner combination. There's no shortage of office furniture available or even basic storage bins.

As with kitchen cabinetry, you're going to want home office storage that doesn't off-gas, has low-maintenance finishes, and is easy to use. Some may offer roll-out shelves, which can make accessing essentials easier. Desktop accessories to keep yourself organized can reduce stress. Now there are also storage cabinets with biometric drawer locks. This is something worth considering to protect the privacy of your important papers.

A home office can double as a library—particularly if you use your books for work reference—with space for a reading lamp and chair. Book lovers will enjoy being surrounded by their favorite volumes during the workday, and floor-to-ceiling bookshelves can reduce noise transference between rooms. A library can also serve as a quiet space in your home when you need a noise or activity break.

LIGHTING

If your work surface is a kitchen island or breakfast bar, it may have existing task lighting. If, on the other hand, it's a desk in a bedroom, it probably does not. The ambient lighting in the room will generally not be enough for a workspace, especially if it's a single lamp in another part of the room or a light fixture centered on the ceiling; that almost guarantees that your upper body will block direct light from shining on your work surface, where it's really needed. If you have a dedicated home office space, task lights installed under a wall cabinet or wall shelf that shine onto your desk are a good alternative to a desk lamp.

Natural light is beneficial for its mood-lifting capabilities but can create glare on computer screens, especially at certain times of day. Being able to enjoy sunshine with diffusion from sheers, blinds, or shades—or a screen protector for your monitor—can give you the best of both worlds.

If your home office doubles as a library, you're going to want lighting that illuminates the shelves, either from the ceiling, the walls, or the bookcases themselves. It won't help your reading habit if it's too dark to find the volume you're seeking.

You might want to consider circadian lighting or smart bulbs if you spend long hours working at home late into the night. It can adjust from bright, cool temperatures in the morning (to get you going) to more relaxed, warm lighting later in the day (to help you shift into relaxing evening mode and sleep later).

TECHNOLOGY

Computers are a fact of work life for most of us. And computers, among other electronics and furnishings, can off-gas toxins into your room. (This is generally in lower amounts than what comes from new cabinetry or carpeting, but it still exists.) Since you may have to use a computer to be productive, keeping the room's air fresh and circulating with an open window, plants, air filtration, and good ventilation is helpful.

For some, the work computer is a laptop that commutes be-tween a home office, vehicle, and traditional workplace. While their portability is a definite advantage, their inflexibility in positioning your hands and eyes ideally at the same time is a definite negative for laptops.

With a separate keyboard and screen, you can set each one at its most ergonomic height for your body. You cannot do that with a laptop, and its constricted screen and keyboard size can create hand and eyestrain.

One option is to take a modular approach to your laptop when working at home. You can use it as a portable information hub while plugging in a separate monitor that can be raised, along with a separate, more ergonomic keyboard and mouse.

Phones are another technology feature of most workplaces, and most health care professionals advise against crimping yours between your neck and shoulder to avoid strain. Headsets can better align your neck. Cordless headsets give you freedom of movement to walk while taking a call. For those counting steps, that can really add to your day's tally, especially if much of your work time is spent on the phone.

There is conflicting information about the dangers of radiation from wireless headphones that can make your workday more productive and ergonomic, and new technologies like the emerging 5G standards will create even more confusion. It's doubtful that you'll be giving up your cell phone, or that your work life would make that even feasible, but how close you want to keep it to your brain is a personal choice. If your work life allows, speakerphone settings may be the safest option until more is known.

One piece of technology that's definitely worth considering for your home office is a shredder. Privacy can become a wellness issue if it's breached, and one way it's done is by people going through your curbside trash and recycling bin. Shredding any mail or paperwork with your name, address, financial account information, and Social Security number helps you avoid becoming an identity thief victim.

Another piece of technology to consider is a speaker for playing your favorite tunes while you work. Mental health professionals say music can help reduce emotional stress and improve well-being.[4]

It can also encourage movement. Get up and dance around your office for a song or two. It will lift your mood and heartbeat.

EXTRAS

Your home office is a great space to reflect your personality. You can celebrate work and other accomplishments with mementos on display. You can include pieces that delight, inspire, or calm you. You can paint the room a relaxing blue or green or a cheerful yellow—just as long as it's low or no VOC paint! If painting isn't an option, you can add color with accessories. The key is to have your office reflect your personality so that you'll enjoy spending many hours working there.

Another option for personal expression is a blackboard or whiteboard. You can use it for doodling, inspiration, memory minders, short-form journaling, or writing love notes to yourself or your partner.

If you have a choice of where to set up your workspace at home, consider a spot with easy access to the outdoors. Anywhere you can take five minutes to enjoy the sunshine on your face, a view to nature, or just a break from being inside can be restorative.

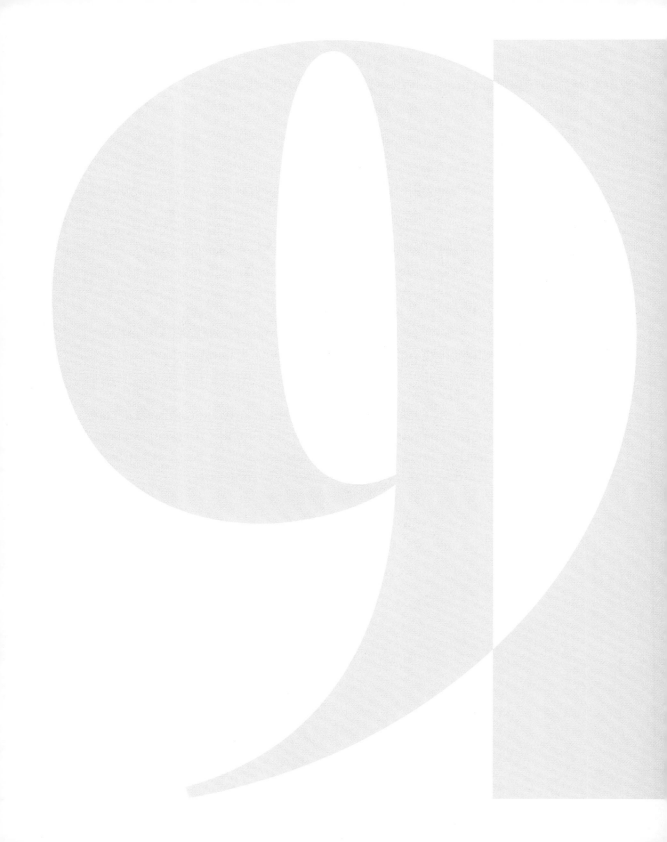

FITNESS SPACE

You want to start an exercise program, but going to a gym isn't practical, perhaps because of a baby or preschooler at home, and running isn't your thing. You still have options, many of them home-friendly. The first step is decide what type of workouts make sense for you and what is involved. And definitely talk to your physician before starting any new workout program.

Your ability and motivation to get started are factors, but so are time, space, and financial commitments. If you're looking at getting into strength training, for example, you're going to need instruction on how to use the equipment safely (ideally with a certified personal trainer), space for a bench and weights, money to buy the gear, and time to train on it.

If spinning is more your style, you'll need the right bike and room to use it. The models that come with built-in training programs tend to be bigger investments. There are numerous cardio-focused and yoga programs that require only room to move, a mat, and a DVD player or Wi-Fi-enabled device. There are also numerous YouTube channels and tablet or mobile phone apps with fitness offerings. Some smart TV systems let you access those through their larger screens for easier visibility.

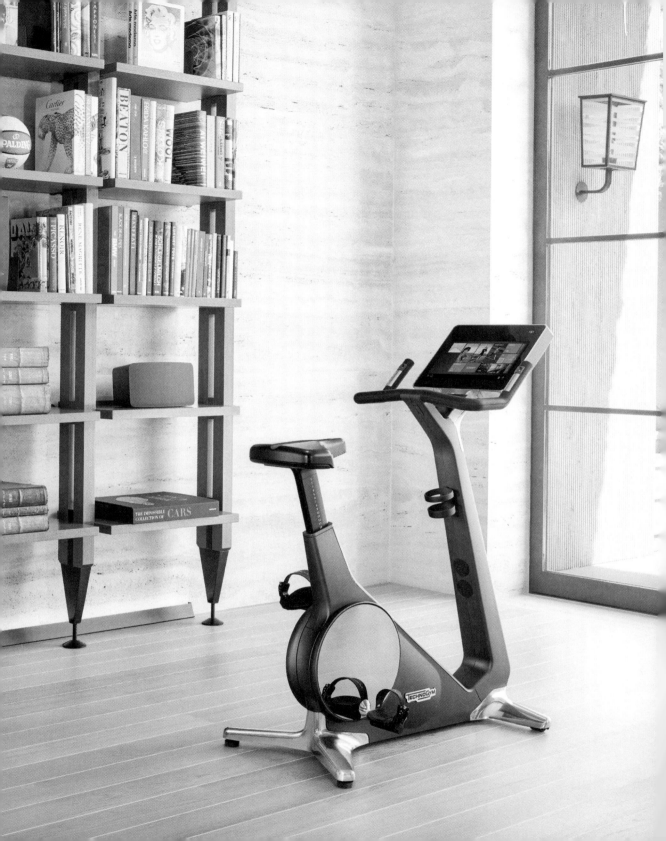

WELLNESS TIP
Light, portable
fitness gear that can
be used anywhere
at home or on the
road is an easy way
to keep fit.

There are also chin-up bars, boxing bags, and suspension systems that can work with your home's existing interior architecture. Suspension workouts have become very popular but can be dangerous if your gear is not properly mounted. Unless your system is portable and designed to take on the road when you travel—as some are—it is vital to have any permanently installed equipment secured to your walls or ceiling properly mounted to studs.

FITNESS AT HOME PLANNING

With any equipment you own or plan to buy, you want to be certain that it's in good condition and set securely in place according to its design specifications. You also want to be sure that you can use your equipment without obstruction or risk to yourself or your home.

It doesn't help to have great gear if it's difficult or unsafe to access. Can you get on and off easily without banging into a wall or large piece of furniture? If it needs to be plugged in, can it be positioned so that the power cord is not in a walk path? If you fall while using it, will you land on something soft or against a hard piece of furniture or a glass window? If you're planning a suspension system, it's ideal to have cushioned slip-resistant mats in place to protect your body and your floors. It's also ideal to have a safe, convenient place for a phone within reach in case you need to call for assistance. These are all considerations to factor into your fitness space planning.

Before bringing large, heavy equipment into a room, like a multi-station gym, make sure that the flooring structure can handle it. This is usually not an issue with a first-floor location on a concrete slab foundation, but it may be planned for a converted attic or second-floor bedroom.

Having exercise equipment at home makes fitness more achievable for even the most time-stressed among us.

You also need to consider vertical clearances. Will running on an elevating treadmill or using a stair climber put your head in the path of a ceiling fan? Given ceiling fans' electrical requirements, you may not have much flexibility in their room placement, so you want to be sure that you have full motion clearance to stay safe.

Some equipment generates noise and/or vibrations. Will it interrupt the sleep or study of anyone on the other side of a wall or directly downstairs? If so, is there a mat you can safely use below it to muffle both noise and vibration? This is especially important for apartment or condo dwellers, parents who can only work out while their young ones are asleep, and couples on split shifts. Your workouts should not be causing sleep interruption or stress to anyone around you.

How much space do your workouts actually require? That's going to vary according to type of workout: Yoga, for example, can be practiced in just a corner of a room, while a full gym may require an entire basement. If you're setting up a workout space in a garage space, you'll find suggestions in chapter 18, "Garage." Privacy can be a factor for workout spaces, both indoors and out, depending on your home's location and seclusion. You don't want strangers or neighbors watching your moves!

You do, however, want to be able to watch yourself work out. This will help you ensure that your form is correct, especially with strength training. Install a wall mirror in your workout space so you can monitor your moves. (Floor mirrors can tip over if you bump into them, so they're not ideal for a workout room.)

THE DEDICATED WORKOUT SPACE

If you're designing a home gym or fitness area from scratch, or completely repurposing a room in your home, you'll also be choosing the flooring materials, lighting, possibly furniture and wall coverings, and athletic equipment you'll need for your workouts.

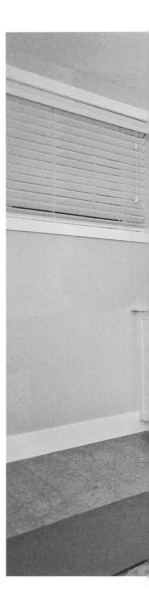

A bar, mirror, and stylish storage help create a welcoming, well-equipped home yoga space.

The room size will be determined by the equipment. If there are space limits, consider what you can best and most safely accommodate. Consider not just how much room the machine itself takes up but how much space is required around it for clearance and how much space you'll need while using it. (For example, a weight bench may be just ten or twelve inches wide, but when you sit on it, your arms and legs will

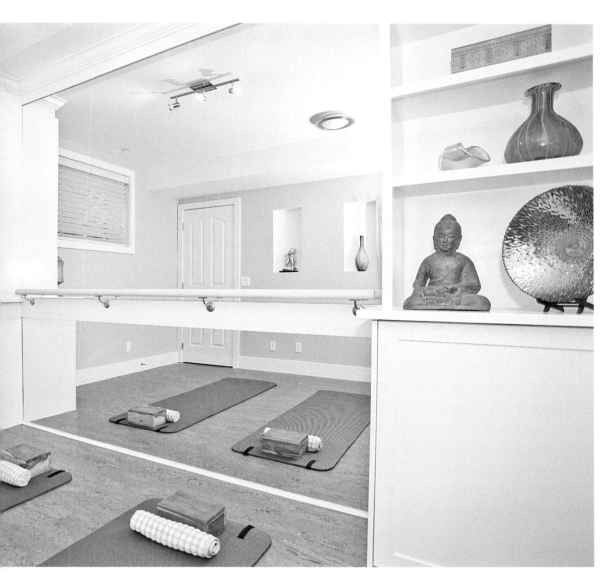

take up extra inches on one or both sides. Make sure you have room to do the exercises, not just place the bench.) Don't overcrowd the room, as you'll end up with an overpriced, under-functioning space.

Different exercise types and equipment also dictate different flooring types. If you're doing high-intensity interval training (HIIT), a surface with some give to it, like cork, rubber, or linoleum, can be kinder to your limbs and joints than concrete or tile.

Most yoga studio owners prefer wood, wood-like bamboo, or laminate as flooring surfaces. These are generally floating floor systems, which have more give than nailed-down wood, concrete, or tile (which also makes them okay for high-impact workouts) while being easy to maintain. Be sure you're choosing a surface without excessive formaldehyde.

Some yoga spaces also incorporate wall bars—or barres, if you prefer. These are great for resistance work and stretching, but must *absolutely, positively* be properly secured. After choosing a comfortable height for your body, be sure to anchor the bars into studs and use rods or dowels that won't give you splinters. If you're going to paint or stain them, go with nontoxic finishes.

A bar alternative can be hooks secured into wall studs for holding exercise bands. They can double as bag or coat hooks when you're not working out, which can be helpful in multipurpose room settings.

When it comes to room paint, you definitely want no- or low-VOC choices. The color will be determined by both your favorite shades and the workout being done. Red or orange can energize—perhaps perfect for your HIIT or spin workout. Blue and green can calm, which may be ideal for your yoga space.

Is noise from the new equipment going to be an issue? Adding soft items like drapes, hanging tapestries, and even houseplants can help. Replacing a hollow-core door with a solid model will also make a difference. If your gym is part of a home addition or down-to-the-studs remodel, you can also have your contractor add insulation to the walls and ceiling.

When considering lighting for your home gym, recessed or flush to the ceiling, so that it doesn't get in the way of your equipment or workouts, is ideal. Dimmable is also preferred, especially when using video. LEDs won't heat up the room the way incandescents used to and use less energy, but if you typically work out in the evening, opt for programmable circadian bulbs so you won't disrupt your sleep cycles.

ESSENTIALS AND EXTRAS

For some equipment, electrical power and protection against weather are necessary. While it's wonderful to run in nature, treadmills require a dry location. They'll handle sweat but not a summer downpour or winter blizzard. If your workout spot isn't weatherized, like a screened-in patio, it may not be feasible for the equipment you want to use.

Good ventilation is also important while you're exercising. If your fitness space is in a garage, you'll either want to keep the door partially open or open a window if there is one. (There's more on garage workout rooms in chapter 18, "Garage.")

If you're using a room in your home, be sure its air filter is clean and the vent is working properly. If you have allergies or asthma, a HEPA filter can be effective in improving your indoor air quality. An air quality monitor is also helpful for an area where you work out, especially if it's located close to a space heater, water heater, pet area, or household cleaner storage space. Your lungs are going to be working hard while you work out. You want to give them the most breathable air possible.

Some equipment should only stand on hard flooring, not carpet, or would likely damage a soft floor like cork or linoleum. Be sure to know the equipment's and floor's specifications before bringing it home.

Is there a spot where you can keep a water bottle within reach? Some pieces of exercise equipment have built-in holders. For machines that don't, where can you stash your hydration so that it's handy but won't get knocked over during your workout? What about a sound speaker or video player for serenading or demonstrating your workout? And where can you store the shoes you need for some workouts? A small storage cabinet or shelf to hold these essentials, along with any other exercise and recovery gear, can be a good use of space. Be sure it's not going to off-gas into the room and it isn't positioned in such a way that you'll slam into it when getting on or off your bike, treadmill, stair climber, or other equipment. A mini-fridge or cold-water dispenser can be a nice add-on to your home gym if you have room in your budget and space.

If the room doesn't have a ceiling fan or central air-conditioning, a window AC unit and standing fan can make strenuous workouts more comfortable. Just as with a cabinet, you'll want to make sure there's plenty of room around a standing fan for your movement and safe passage. If this isn't possible, a table fan on top of a storage cabinet can make good use of limited space.

WELLNESS TIP
Set up a digital picture frame to hold inspirational images in view while you work out. These can be changed to provide timely goal motivation for different training programs.

SWIM SPAS

Swimming and water aerobics—covered in chapter 6, "Outdoor Living Spaces"—are great low-impact exercises.[1] Many coaches and physical therapists recommend hydrotherapy for reducing muscle tension, for pain relief, as a low-impact alternative to running when tendinitis or other injuries strike, and for overall stress relief. If you don't have access to an all-season gym or community pool, or room to add one at your home, a swim spa (or fitness pool) is a possible solution.

Like traditional spas, swim spas circulate warm water, but they're focused more on movement than on sitting. Consider them swimming treadmills. You're moving against a jet-generated current in a fitness pool. You can adjust the current's speed, just as you can adjust a treadmill's speed, and get your laps completed without needing a twenty-five- or fifty-meter pool for a good workout.

Just as with treadmills, there are bells and whistles you can add to your swim spa, depending on your budget. Some offer seats for relaxation and socializing, as well as speakers for your workout tunes or app routines, mirrors to observe your form, and stairs with handrails for safer entry and exit. They vary in size—from seven or eight feet by ten feet for a compact model to more than twenty feet, often with their own separate seated spa. The recommended size for effective swimming workouts is in the twelve-to-sixteen-foot range.

Some swim spas are designed for interior-only use and some are rated for outdoor environments; be sure to get the right type for your planned setting. While less expensive than a traditional built-in pool, swim spas are still an investment; it's worth spending time talking to a swim coach and/or a reputable dealer (perhaps referred by a coach) before selecting and installing one. There are portable models—also called self-contained or prebuilt—that you can take with you when you move. If this is a consideration, you'll definitely want to ask about what's available when you shop for yours.

HOUSE CALL

It is a mistake to think of exercise as an optional part of your week. It is as important for good health as brushing your teeth, showering, and getting a good night's rest. By physically challenging yourself through exercise, you strengthen your ability to be disciplined, impose at least a small amount of structure into the week, reduce anxiety, impose a bulwark against depression, enhance confidence, and reduce stress. If exercise came in a pill form, its beneficial properties would be considered magical.
—*Forrest Talley, PhD, psychologist, Folsom, California; forresttalley.com*

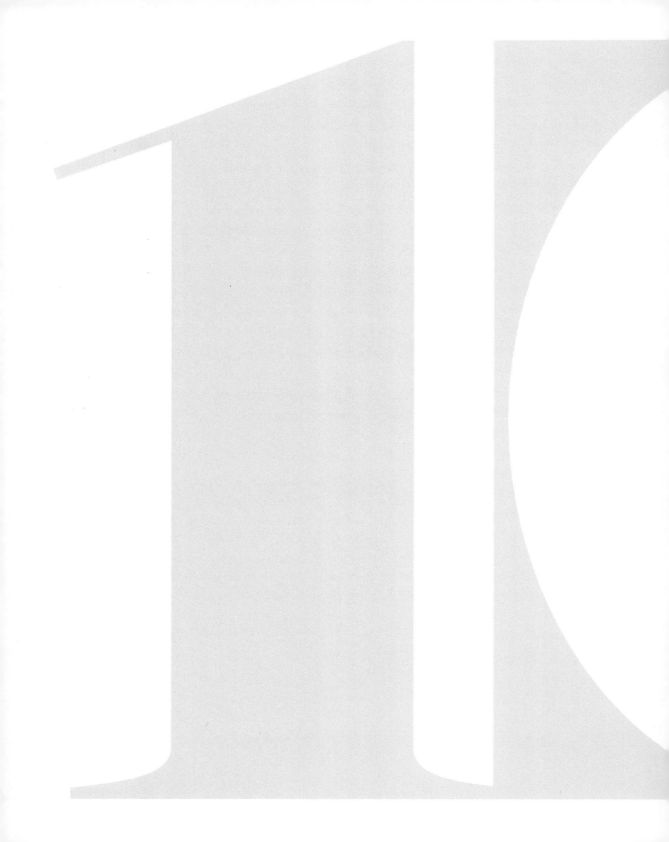

Public LIVING SPACES

What makes a room "public"? This generally applies to spaces in your home where you spend time with friends, family, and other guests for social activities. These would include your great room, dining room, and rec room. Contrast these with your master bedroom and bathroom, where your purpose is sleep and hygiene, or with your home office, where your purpose is work.

The public areas of your home are for gathering and relaxing. Your entries and powder room are also public spaces, in the sense that they'll be used by guests, as well as the home's residents, but they're not gathering places. Let's look at enhancing the wellness of these areas, for your household's and your guests' benefit as well as your own.

CREATING HEALTHIER SPACES

The more your home connects to the nature outside its walls, the easier it is to create healthy living spaces. If you're building or remodeling, position as many doors and windows as you can to

take advantage of breezes, views, and easy access to your outdoor areas. Many houses today are designed for indoor-outdoor
living, with entertaining areas divided solely by walls of retracting
glass doors. Not only does this create fabulous flow for your gather-
ings, it can also reduce the amount of recycled air you have to
breathe.

Another wellness strategy is to build or add only the square
footage your household really needs, so that you're not spending
time and money maintaining rooms you'll rarely use. Opting for
low-maintenance materials, even in your "show" spaces, is similarly
beneficial: You'll have more time and money left over for exploring the
national parks or traveling abroad for your dream race.

You can also devote more of your public entertaining space to
outdoor activities like grilling or playing sports and games together
rather than sitting inside and watching TV. The less your living space
is designed around a television, the more active and social you'll find
your time spent at home to be.

Another wellness strategy is to design all of your areas to be
accessible by—and hospitable to—anyone visiting your home with
mobility challenges. After all, an injury could impact you at some
point, too, and you could find yourself seriously inconvenienced in
your own home temporarily. This includes having a powder room that
someone in a wheelchair can use as easily as anyone else. (That's easier
to accomplish for new construction projects than when you're remodeling, unless you have space you can borrow from an adjacent room.)

If you're building or improving your "forever" dream home to
spend your golden years in, and it's a multilevel residence, it's worth
considering adding an elevator. One can be added later—especially if
the space is planned accordingly, often with closets "stacked" on upper

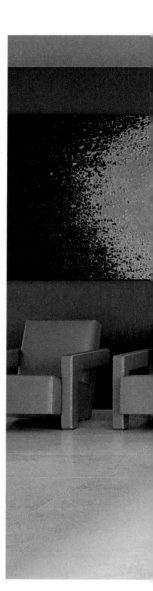

*Walls that open wide
with stacking doors and
outdoor-rated porcelain
tiles make indoor-
outdoor living easy.*

and lower floors—but it's easiest for a new build. Given the cost of land in many parts of the country, two- and three-story homes make more sense—and are easier to find than single stories—but can be tough for someone who has trouble climbing or descending stairs. If you've ever run an ultramarathon or completed a twenty-four-hour rucking event, you might find that applies to you as well!

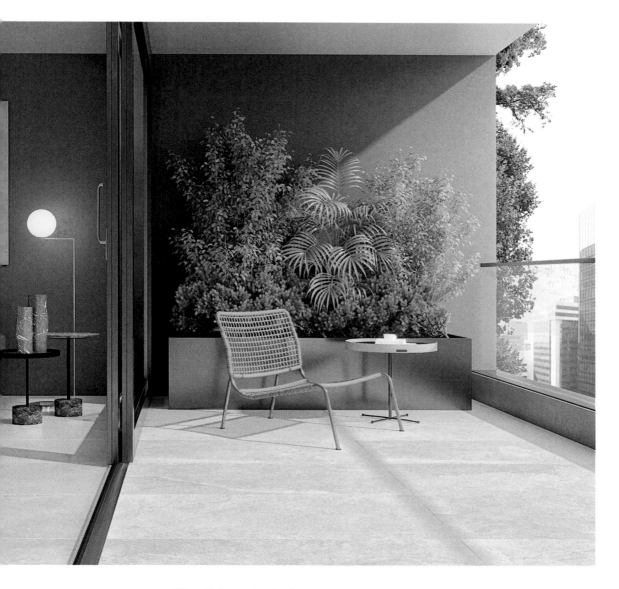

DINING ROOMS

Your dining area may be completely open to your kitchen and other living areas, indoors and out. That's becoming increasingly common in the most popular floor plans. Dining areas need their own lighting, especially if they're used for other purposes, like studying or work. This can be recessed lighting, track lighting, or fixtures—whichever works best for the space's ceiling structure and design. While the room may have its own ambient lighting—often from large windows and recessed ceiling cans—the dining table should have its own task lighting. That can be a single large fixture or a series of two or three, depending on size. A general rule of thumb is thirty inches between hanging lights, so a six-foot dining table would have two.

Any space where knives are used should be well lit, but a dimming capacity is ideal for creating relaxation at the table with softer illumination. An increasingly popular feature for lighting is automation, whether by voice control, programmed themes, or both. (It's fun to be able to tell your app to "entertain" and have those lights warm and dim, the shades come down, and soft music play.) Circadian lighting tied into your smart home system will let you enjoy crisp, bright light in the morning as you're getting ready for your day with coffee and breakfast, and a calming glow for dinner—all programmed into the lighting system.

Dining tables can be made of a wide range of materials, from wood to porcelain to glass to metal to stone. Consider which surface's maintenance requirements best fit your lifestyle, as you and your household will be using and cleaning the tabletop multiple times a day. If you have young children or large, boisterous pets, consider whether spilled beverages will have a damaging impact on your table if not quickly addressed. (The discussion of countertops in chapter 3, "Material Choices," will help you decide on table surfaces too.)

The shape of your table will be determined by the room's size, but you definitely want to allow enough space to walk around it so someone can get up from a seat without banging into a wall or a piece of furniture. This is generally considered to be thirty-six inches, except at room entryways, where you will want at least forty-eight inches and preferably sixty.

If you have toddlers or seniors in the home or as regular guests, consider whether rounded corners might be the safer option to offset falls. Another recent trend is the bar table. These thirty-six- or forty-two-inch-high pieces for standing at while using, or sitting at on stools, are admittedly helpful in cramped spaces and on small balconies, but they can make it harder to use for someone who has balance or mobility issues, and can be uncomfortable for someone shorter in stature. That's definitely something to consider for seniors, who are more likely to suffer falls.

If you enjoy spending long hours at the dinner table, consider the comfort of your dining chairs. There isn't a one-size-fits-all solution, so it's best to try out seating before you purchase, if possible. Back support is ideal, as is some cushioning. There are many classic chair styles with bare wood backs and seats. You may love their look, but consider how comfortable they'll feel by the dessert course of a dinner party or game night.

One of the challenges with fabrics and fillers is toxicity. Some of the low-maintenance materials that make furniture stain-resistant and cleanup easier can also make you sick. (Those with chemical sensitivities will feel it first, but there are potential lasting effects for individuals without chemical sensitivities as well.) Machine-washable fabrics or leather treated without toxins are healthier options.

LIVING ROOMS AND GREAT ROOMS

Whatever your space is called—living or great room—it's largely designed for socializing and relaxing. This area is often open to the kitchen and dining areas, which is wonderful for parties but not necessarily ideal for weight management, as your pantry and refrigerator may be in open view and easy reach of your television viewing with all of its food ads.

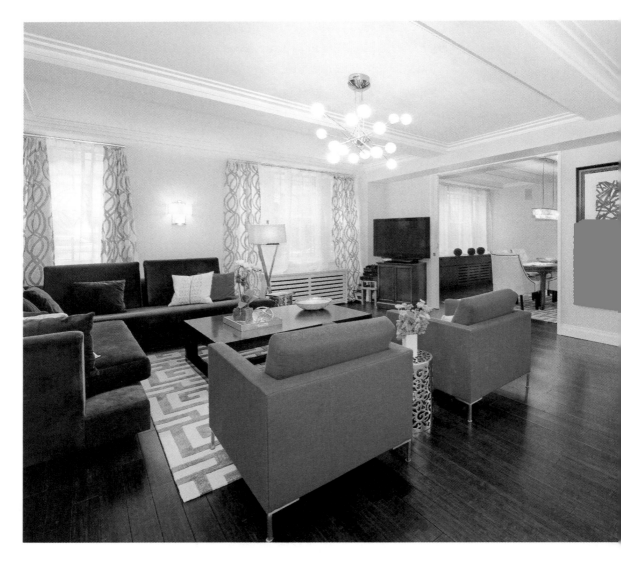

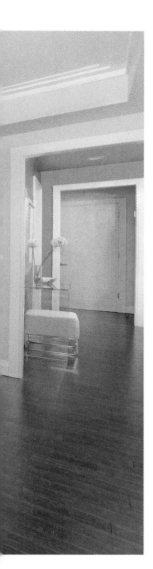

If your willpower is weak—and most people's is!—you can orient your furniture so that your seating is facing away from the kitchen. You could, of course, locate your favorite TV in another room a flight of stairs away from the kitchen if possible. (Might the increasing size of our waistlines relate to the increasing size of our TVs, their appetite-driving commercials, the easy proximity of our pantries and refrigerators, and the increasing number of hours we spend on our couches?)

The furniture filling your living space will reflect your taste. It can also reflect your household for more livability. If you have two black Labrador retrievers, a black leather couch (or machine washable dark couch cover) will be much easier to live with than light-colored, dry-clean-only upholstery.

If you have young children or animals, a fabric you can easily spot treat, like denim or chenille, or kid- and pet-tolerant leather will be more family-friendly than worrying that they're ruining an expensive, delicate piece. (You know this already, but it's tempting sometimes to indulge in trends.) If you get distressed leather seating, it will be easier to hide damage by two- and four-legged family members.

Just as with your dining table, consider rounded, softened edges for coffee tables and perhaps avoid glass or marble. An ottoman is a good, soft alternative, and one with storage will provide a good spot for toys when they're not in use. (This also eliminates a trip hazard in your home.)

Living areas often have lamps and rugs. Both can add great style but can be trip hazards as well. With lamps, it's the cord that's likely to be the problem. If you can position the lamp so that the cord is against a wall and not crossing an area with foot traffic, that will eliminate its potential to trip someone. If that's not possible, place the lamp where it will provide the light needed for reading or crafts but where its cord

Furniture made without toxic materials is ideal for those with chemical sensitivities and overall healthier home spaces.

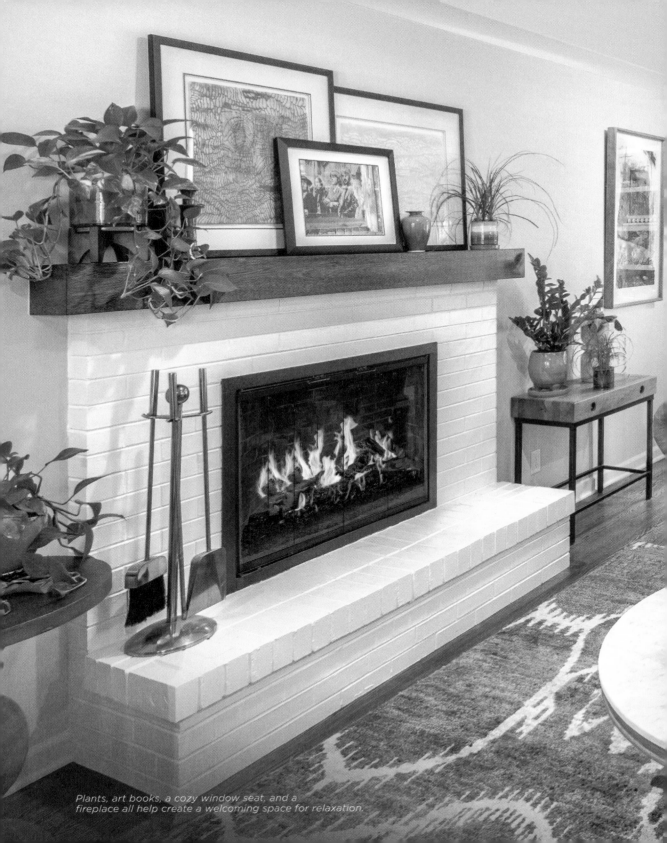

Plants, art books, a cozy window seat, and a fireplace all help create a welcoming space for relaxation.

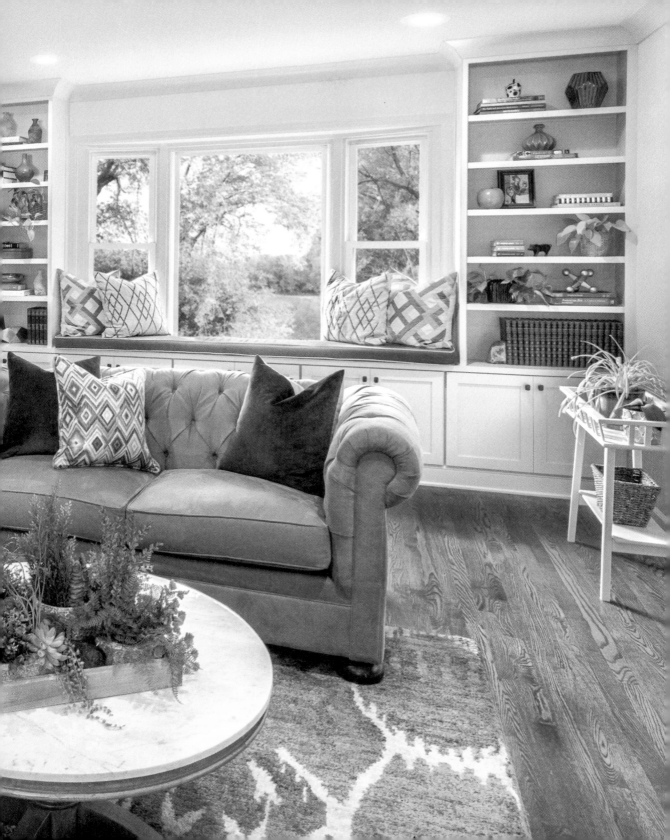

won't cross a busy path. If neither is doable, consider having an electrician wire a ceiling pendant, so no cords will be needed at all!

Rugs soften a room, but their edges can also be a trip hazard, especially for seniors. A gripper system can keep them in place and protect your floor. You can find nontoxic rugs in an online search or in designer boutiques. They're likely to be wool, natural fibers (like sisal or seagrass), or recycled materials.

Living area flooring may be carpeted, wood, laminate, bamboo, tile, or another hard surface. If you're looking to replace what's covering yours now, chapter 3, "Material Choices," will provide all of the properties, positive and negative, of each. Hard surfaces tend to be favored by those with pets, kids, and/or allergies. People with chemical sensitivities may want to consider tile instead of an engineered surface. It can look like wood, stone, or even fabric, and won't off-gas. Area rugs can warm and soften hard floors.

Great rooms and living rooms are typically where you'll find the household's main television. The big screen is where you gather for the big game or family movies. It's date night central for you and your partner. These days your TV is likely to sit on a low cabinet or be mounted to a wall. If it sits on a piece of furniture and you have children, be sure to secure it in place so that it can't be pulled down on top of an unsuspecting child.

Height matters for comfortable viewing, especially if you're going to binge-watch. Commercials might be a pain in the neck; you don't want watching your favorite show to be one too. You generally want the center of the screen to be at eye level. That might differ for two users, but you can make an average between you work.

It's not uncommon to find a TV mounted over a fireplace. Given the latter's height and clearance requirements, that might be too high for comfortable viewing. A mount that angles the screen toward the viewer or even lowers the screen can be helpful for avoiding neck strain.

While the TV may be the focal point of your living area, there are benefits to adding art that personalizes the space for you. (There are now television sets that can display your favorite photos or paintings digitally when you're not watching a show; this is definitely a personalized option worth considering.)

This is where you'll spend time relaxing with a favorite book, craft, family member, or friend. Displaying decorative elements that delight or inspire you adds to your mental well-being while you enjoy your living spaces.

Plants are also great additions to these public areas in your home. They create a welcoming environment, become an attractive visual element, lift your mood, and enhance your indoor air quality, a decided benefit to a space with off-gassing electronics like televisions. (The degree to which plants can improve air quality varies by type, light levels, room size and ventilation, and other factors.)

HOUSE CALL

In our stress management program, participants put house plants on their desks and received fun texts prescribing time outside and mindfulness. These indoor and outdoor nature elements, along with easy reset-your-breathing techniques, prove helpful in reversing the effects of work-related burnout.
—Dr. John La Puma, MD, FACP, founder of A Green Rx, Santa Barbara, California; drjohnlapuma.com

DENS AND STUDIES

These are often designed as quiet spaces in the home. A couch, comfy reading chair, or day bed make this a restful room. Cabinetry to hold books, photos, and collectibles can surround you with treasured memories and reduce noise. (Look for nontoxic storage that won't fill your retreat with chemical fumes!)

If you'll use this room for long hours, perhaps to study for a class or enjoy your favorite novel, an ergonomic armchair that supports your back and neck while you read or relax will be ideal. You'll also want a task light near that chair to shed light on your book or project. A wool area rug adds natural softness to hard flooring, or visual interest to wall-to-wall carpeting. Consider a gripper pad in either case so that no one trips on its edges or corners, yourself included.

If the room's layout allows for it to be closed off, your den or study can become a quiet retreat. French doors can keep it connected to the rest of the home. Closable blinds or drapery panels mounted on them can give you privacy and darkness for an afternoon recharging nap. Everyone needs downtime on occasion; a den or study can be the home space that provides it with comfort, inspiration, and joy.

GAME AND REC ROOMS

At the other end of the spectrum are busy game or rec rooms. These are a home's let-loose areas, often filled with kids or teens. They should be as low-maintenance as possible, with durable finishes.

Distressed wood, tile, or linoleum are all good flooring options. You can stain a concrete floor, perhaps giving it a playful, personalized design inspired by your favorite sport, team, trip, or memory. (You can always cover it with another material later if you decide to sell the house.)

Nontoxic carpet tiles are another good option, especially in a basement space that is often naturally colder, or one used by young children and toddlers. Always buy extra, so you can more easily replace a damaged tile later. A wall covered in chalkboard paint or a whiteboard is convenient for keeping score during games and can provide a creativity outlet.

Sturdy distressed, nontoxic leather furniture is easy to clean and long-lasting. Also, look for used pieces you won't worry about getting damaged. Washable slipcovers are helpful, too, but may be dragged out of place regularly by active kids.

Game tables are great for getting kids—and grown-ups—off the

If your rec room is in a basement, consider adding a radon detector, as basements are more prone to this serious, invisible, odor-free pollutant in the soil all around us. A radon detector will also make it a more worry-free space.

couch. Consider games that involve the most movement, like table tennis. Video systems that get you dancing or doing yoga or high-intensity workouts are great too. The idea is to create an indoor space that encourages active socialization or fitness for yourself.

Game and rec rooms often have bars or mini-kitchens, but these don't have to promote unhealthy habits. A mini-fridge can hold water instead of soda, and healthier snacks for your young athletes. Consider an air popper instead of a microwave.

Whether you make your rec room the TV watching zone is up to you. On the one hand, it makes your upstairs living area more about socializing than screen time. On the other hand, it moves the TV to the space where your kids will be spending the most time. If you want to limit their watching, this might not be your best option.

If your hobby involves souvenir mugs, sports memorabilia, or other sentimental collectibles, a rec room is a great place to display those. You'll certainly want to keep them away from small reaching hands or from the arc of a billiard ball potentially heading their way! Shelving high up on the wall and museum wax to keep them in place can be a good option.

It's not uncommon to see a game or rec room double as a man cave. If that's how yours will be used, consider adding a beer tap, wine fridge, and/or coffee station for adult refreshment. A man cave would call for a good couch; again, distressed, nontoxic leather is a great option for low maintenance, hard-used living areas—and a place for the guys to put their feet up on a sturdy coffee table while watching the big game.

Rec rooms don't necessarily need task lighting, but ambient lighting on a dimmer is helpful. If the space is being used for TV or movie watching, you'll want to be able to block out external light. If it's being used for yoga or fitness, you'll want to block out external views for privacy. Any space in your home designed for adult, child, or teen playtime should be stress-free, worry-free, and filled with fun.

POWDER AND REC ROOM BATHROOMS

When you can make these accessible with wider doorways and grab bars, you'll have a more usable, accessible, and valuable home. Even if widening doorways isn't a short-term option, you can still select a taller comfort-height toilet that's easier to get on and off of— something you'll also appreciate after an endurance event—and add grab bars combined with shelves, toilet paper holders, or towel bars flanking it. The shelf models can double as phone and purse holders without detracting from the style of the room. A hook on the back of the door or a side wall for coats or shoulder bags is also a convenience for users so they don't have to fumble with them or place them on the floor—no one's favorite option.

Making a bathroom accessible and safer enhances your home's value and "visitability."

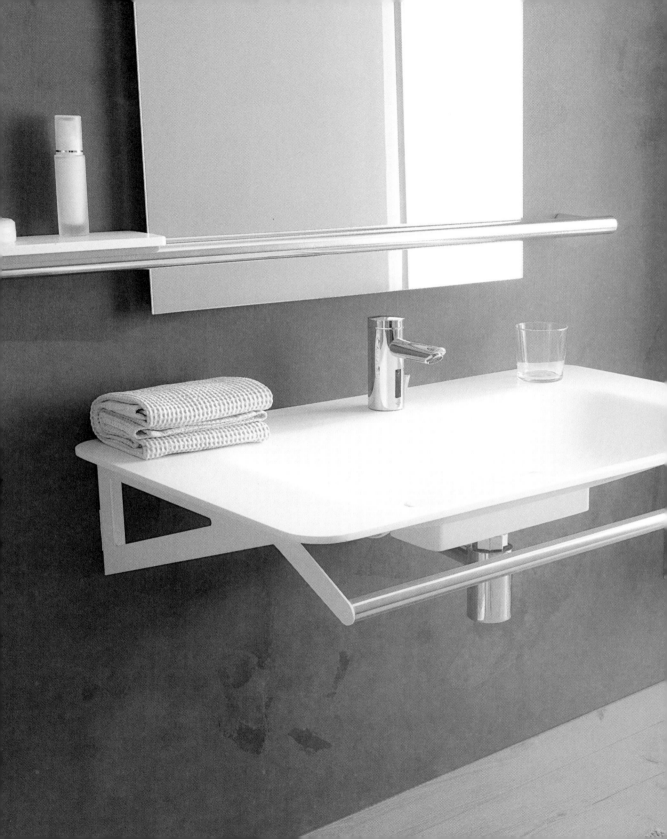

MASTER BEDROOM

We spend almost a third of our lives sleeping, so the space where it happens can have a tremendous impact on our well-being. It's not uncommon to have times in your life when worry keeps you awake, but if not getting enough quality sleep is a common occurrence, there are ways to improve your bedroom that can possibly make a difference.

Before doing so, it makes sense to consult with your doctor to see if there are physical or mental health issues that need to be addressed. He or she may suggest a prescription, over-the-counter sleep supplement, stress reduction techniques, or reducing your use of electronics before bedtime, as their blue light has been shown to interfere with sleep. If you're ready for the next step, let's look at your bedroom itself and how it can be redesigned to support your need for quality sleep.

Sleep is the time when your body repairs itself. If you do not get enough sleep, your body's ability to repair even normal day-to-day damage is compromised. Sleep deprivation interferes with memory, impairs immune function, and interrupts the body's hormones and neurotransmitters—your brain's silent instructions to your heart, lungs, and stomach to function properly. The impact is really to every single cell in the body. It's almost impossible to be a healthy individual if you're not getting good, restful sleep.

—Dr. David Leopold, MD, DABFM, DABOIM, network medical director of Hackensack Meridian Integrative Health & Medicine, Red Bank, New Jersey; hackensackmeridianhealth.org

WINDOW COVERINGS

Natural light is ideal for creating a welcoming space—including enjoying your bedroom on the rare morning when you can luxuriate in bed or cuddle there with your partner or kids—but a full moon shining into your windows at night may not be conducive to sleep. Neither is a streetlight, the headlights from passing cars, or the glare

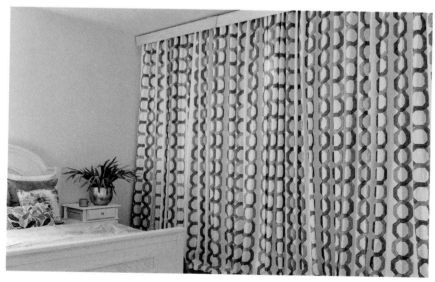

Blackout panels block outside lights for better sleep.

of a neighborhood watch volunteer's flashlight beaming into your room. Any of these can keep sleep at bay or even wake you up in the middle of the night.

Blackout drapery panels, blackout liners for standard drapes, or properly mounted blackout shades will greatly reduce the chance of outdoor lights interrupting your sleep. Panels and liners (used with standard drapes) cover the entire window, blocking out all external light. They also give you more design flexibility, as you can choose whatever type of blinds or shades appeal to your taste, and darken the room completely by closing the panels.

Shades need to be very carefully measured so that they don't allow in light if they're mounted within the window frame, as is often the case. Otherwise, their room-darkening potential will be limited by the narrow sliver of light slicing through.

Don't forget about covering a bathroom window if that space is open to the bedroom. You may be restricted to moisture-friendly blinds if the window is in the shower stall, but unless the window is in direct view of the bedroom or very close, a blind should address most room-darkening needs. (The bigger sleep issue with open master suite layouts is having a couple on different schedules sharing the space.)

LIGHTING

Energy-efficient lighting is great for saving money on your utility bills and saving the planet. It isn't great for your sleep, though, as it often contains high levels of blue light, which research shows to have negative effects on your body's ability to produce its sleep hormone.[1]

There are energy-efficient LED bulbs designed with reduced blue light that are ideal for bedside lamps and ceiling fixtures. There is also circadian technology for smart home lighting that shifts from a brighter, bluer spectrum by day to a warmer, softer spectrum at night. This may be an excellent option for your bedroom's lighting sources, be they chandeliers, pendants, sconces, lamps, or recessed lights. All can be tied to a home automation system you can program to ease yourself from daytime to sleep time.

ELECTRONICS

Don't disregard the light from the electronics in your bedroom. Many cable boxes, TVs, and clock radios have light indicators on their faces; if those are blue, they, too, can interrupt your sleep. There are also alarm clocks that wake you up with soft light, rather than sound, for a more natural, less jarring start to your day. TV, tablet, and smartphone screens can have a potentially even larger effect, and sleep experts recommend not having any of them in your bedroom if you have consistent insomnia issues,[2] and turning them off two to three hours before bed in any case.[3] If checking your phone, laptop, or tablet before bed is important to you, consider using an app that shifts their screens to circadian lighting.

If you need to see the face of your clock radio, choose one with red numbers instead of blue. Some new televisions offer blue-light filters as well. If you absolutely can't go to sleep without your dose of late-night comedy and a filter isn't feasible for you, get as much bright light as you can during the day to offset your TV's blue-light effects at night.

Televisions and other electronics can also off-gas, releasing toxic dust into your home's atmosphere. Air purifiers and houseplants can offset their impact to a certain extent; if you're ultrasensitive to chemicals, it may be better not to have a TV in your bedroom at all, considering how much time you spend there.

As mentioned, an air purifier is an electronic purchase worth considering for your bedroom. It can pull impurities out of the environment so you're not breathing them in while you sleep. These can include pet dander; secondhand smoke from a neighbor; car exhaust from a nearby road; mold and pollen; and toxins from your home environment. A model with a HEPA filter will be the most effective. It won't remove irritants from surfaces like bedding, carpets, rugs, or drapes, but it will capture those floating in the room's air.

WELLNESS TIP
If your TV doesn't have a blue-light filter feature, you can purchase and add a screen to accomplish the same goal.

Some people can't sleep in an absolutely quiet room. A white-noise machine or phone app might work for these individuals. The machine with a non–blue-light power indicator is probably a better bet than the phone app, as it won't interrupt your sleep with late-night texts, distract you with social media notifications, or send email alerts at odd hours. Alternatively, a ceiling fan, an air purifier, the click of blinds against the frame of an open window on a breezy night, or the soft chirp of crickets outside might be all the sound you need.

NOISE

Noise can be a problem for sleep and relaxation, especially in apartment and condo buildings, but if it's coming from outside, you may not be able to eliminate it with a neighborly conversation. Rugs, drapes, a solid-core door, nontoxic sound-deadening paints and wall coverings, and even tall cabinetry can muffle sound on the other side of a wall, and ceiling fans and white-noise machines can camouflage them. Weather stripping around your doors and windows can reduce the amount of noise that seeps into your home from outside when they're closed. So can adding cabinetry on a wall with noisy neighbors. Books can insulate sound, and glass doors will keep them from collecting allergy-spurring dust. A clothing wardrobe or linen cabinet can do the same. If your bed is against a noisy wall, or too close to a noisy room in your own home, consider moving it to another area of the room if possible.

Leafy houseplants can also help absorb noise. When choosing one for your bedroom, be sure to ask your local plant specialist what will grow best with your bedroom's light levels and not present a hazard to your pets if they're allowed into the space.

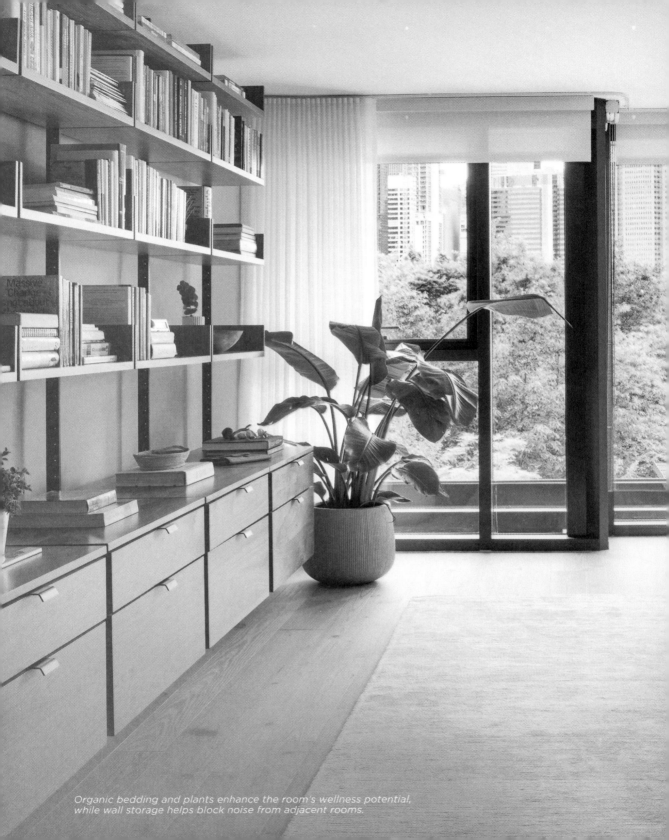

Organic bedding and plants enhance the room's wellness potential, while wall storage helps block noise from adjacent rooms.

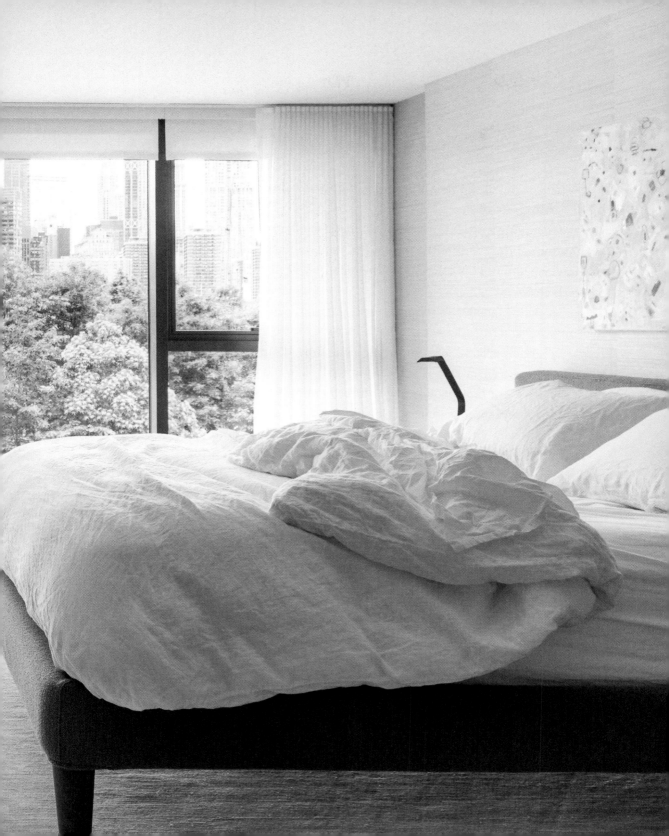

CLIMATE

Part of sleeping comfortably is having the right temperature and humidity levels in your room. Most health experts consider sixty to sixty-seven degrees Fahrenheit to be the ideal temperature level for adult sleep.[4] If it's too hot or cold, you could have a harder time falling asleep or be woken out of slumber more easily. Neither is ideal for getting a full, restful night of sleep.

Installing a programmable thermostat can help you find the right temperature within that range and then set it to adjust during your sleep hours. This can provide the ideal sleep temperature for your bedroom.

A ceiling fan helps a room feel cooler from the movement of air around you and provides white noise. Since it can also move dust and other allergens around the room at the same time, it's important to keep the blades clean. It's also important to sleep in a location that doesn't direct the fan's cooling power directly onto your body. That can result in muscle soreness and skin irritation if you're prone to dryness.

If you're in a very dry climate, a humidifier can also help you sleep more comfortably. Health pros say humidifiers reduce snoring; ease dry skin, throat, lips, eyes, and hair; relieve allergies and sinus headaches; and possibly even help you avoid catching the flu.[5] In order to be a health benefit, though, humidifiers need to be checked and cleaned regularly. If you're having temporary or ongoing respiratory issues, check with your doctor about whether you should be using one. You can also ask your doctor what type of humidifier would be best for your health.

MATTRESSES AND PILLOWS

As anyone who has ever spent a night on the ground during a back-packing trip or multiday trail run can tell you, what's beneath your body when you sleep can have a tremendous impact on how you feel when you wake up. For most of us at home, that's a mattress. Is yours ready to be replaced? If you wake up with lower back pain every day that is not related to another physical condition, it could be time for a new mattress.

Choosing one is no small feat, especially with the overwhelming level of selections available, but choosing well is vitally important. Consider that you'll spend almost a third of your next decade on it and you'll realize that it's worth the investment of time and money to buy one that's right for you. (It's also a home-related investment you can take with you when you move, so it works for tenants as well as homeowners.)

The first thing to know is that one-size-fits-all does not apply to mattress types. You want one that supports your body in the positions in which you habitually sleep. For some, that's the side; for others, the back or stomach. If you have the chance to check out mattresses in person and spend some quality time on them, that will be a good indicator. Many companies that don't sell through retail showrooms offer a trial period with a money-back guarantee.

Innerspring mattresses, the most common type you'll find at mattress stores, offer good support but can contain toxins that off-gas. If you go with this option, be sure to let it air out for as long as necessary outside of your bedroom before you start sleeping on it.

Adjustable beds can be a good choice for individuals with sleep apnea, acid reflux, or mobility issues that make it harder to sit up. Memory foam mattresses have gotten popular in recent years, as they mold to your body while supporting it, and can be helpful for couples sharing a bed. But they can also make you feel warmer at night, and some emit chemical fumes.

There are mattresses made of all-natural materials like undyed wool that won't off-gas for healthier sleep, but they are only available from specialty sources at a higher cost. To persuade you to make the investment, many of their manufacturers offer free trial periods and money-back guarantees.

Pillows are also essential for comfortable, healthier sleep, and are also individualistic. Some people love the natural softness of down, while others are allergic to the feathers or want a more moldable foam, but without toxic elements. Side sleepers have different needs than back or stomach sleepers, and there are pillows catering to each. The key for any pillow is to support your neck in a neutral position so it doesn't feel sore when you wake up.

Whichever position you sleep in, choosing a pillow with a natural covering and filling will give you a healthier night's sleep. Organic wool and cotton, natural latex, and foam are all good options. Many companies make comfort claims, and being able to return a pillow that doesn't live up to your expectations is ideal. You want pillows that are both comfortable and natural so that you can breathe easily through the night.

BEDDING

Natural bedding made from cotton, linen, hemp, wool, or bamboo, and washed regularly with a natural detergent, is ideal for a sleeping environment. For allergy sufferers, bedrooms can be especially difficult areas, medical specialists say, as so many hours are spent there, and dust mites often inhabit beds and bedding.[6] Covering your mattress and pillows with natural fabric covers and using hot water at least every week or two to wash all your bedding can reduce levels of allergens and other irritants.

In addition to sheets and pillowcases, you can find natural duvets, duvet covers, and throws. Taking a layered approach to your bedding can help you find a comfort level for sleep and adjust as needed without changing the thermostat. Layering can also keep relations healthier between partners with different internal temperatures. If you're most comfortable at sixty-five degrees and your partner is most comfortable at sixty, you can cover yourself with a throw while he or she uses only a top sheet or light duvet.

STORAGE

Bedroom storage needs generally include clothing, shoes, possibly
jewelry, and a few personal items you like having close at hand at
night—perhaps a rope ladder for an upper-floor emergency escape and
a flashlight with extra batteries for safety; a phone charger; and a book.
Clothing will take up the greatest amount of space, and the more or-
ganization you can create with your garments, the less time and stress
will be involved with finding what you need—especially on race days or
before important work events.

If you're limited to a single standard closet, consider storing
just what you wear most often there and adding under-bed storage
or a wardrobe for other clothing. Your workout or yoga clothes that
don't wrinkle can have their own space in an easy-to-reach under-
bed bin, and your special occasion outfits that get worn less often can
hang in a spare bedroom closet if you have one, or in the back of the
closet if you don't.

If you're adding cabinetry to your bedroom, be sure to choose
pieces without formaldehyde and toxic finishes. You don't want to be
breathing those toxins all night. If you go with taller units, a pull-down
closet rod will help you maximize your space and increase its accessibility. Many experienced racers lay out their clothes and shoes the
night before, but you don't want to struggle to find what you'll need
when you really want to get some extra sleep.

Even if you're not remodeling your closet, you can add a valet
hook to hang the next day's garments and avoid stress in the morning.
That will help you get to your meeting or the starting line of your half
marathon faster and more relaxed.

MORNING KITCHENS

People with larger multistory homes sometimes have morning kitchens adjacent to their master bedrooms and bathrooms. A morning kitchen is an add-on area where cold drinks can be kept chilled, snacks and coffee can be prepared, and wine can be stored and served, depending on the homeowners' tastes. It can also hold a few place settings and possibly a compact dishwasher.

A master suite with this amenity is also likely to have a sitting room or balcony, so that drinks chilled in the beverage fridge or poured from a coffee system can be enjoyed in private at the start or end of the day.

If privacy and relaxation are wellness features—and one can definitely make the case that they are—a morning kitchen and sitting areas are premium wellness spaces worth considering for your life and home.

A morning kitchen adds the potential for breakfast in bed or a glass of wine after work to your master suite.

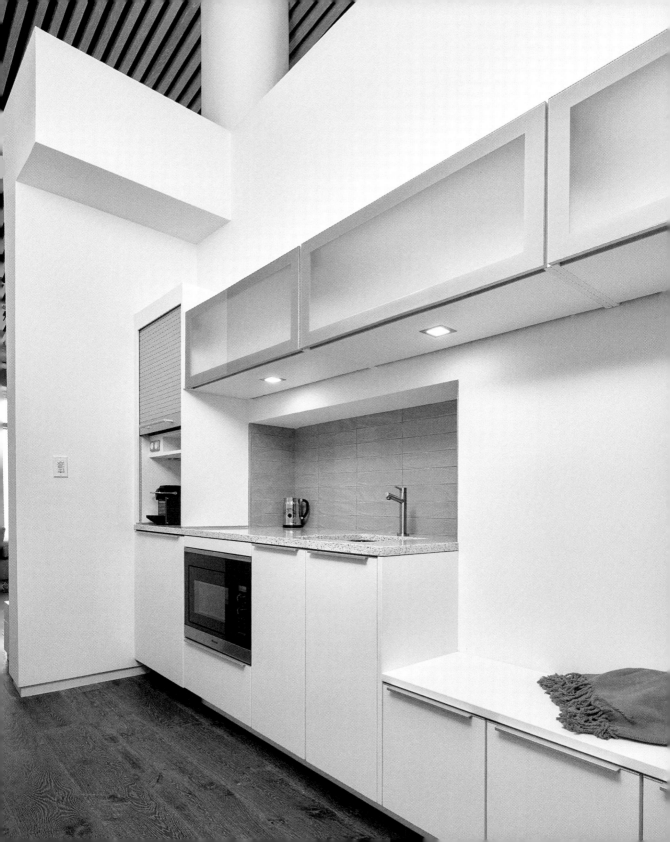

MASTER BATHROOM

If you live in a single-family home built in the last two decades, you probably have a bathroom within your master suite, used only by you and possibly a significant other. If you're in the process of buying a home, even a condo or town house, the size and amenities offered in those precious square feet will greatly influence how much you'll enjoy—and pay for—the property. (An apartment with a spacious, well-appointed master bath will also likely be more expensive to rent.) After the kitchen, the master bath is probably the most important consideration in a home-buying decision. As well it should be!

The master bath is where we start our day and where we get ready for bed every night. It's also where we shower or bathe after our workouts, brush our teeth, shave, do our makeup, and attend to bodily needs. This is prime real estate in our daily lives, as well as in the value of our homes. It can also be prime real estate for our wellness. The master bath can impact our safety, health, work and athletic performance, schedules, recovery, and comfort.

These can be enhanced not only by what's in the room but how it's laid out. The good news is that many of today's popular design trends are naturally beneficial to our well-being. This wasn't always the case. In past years, master baths included polished stone floors and palatial steps leading up to grandiose bathtubs. Both represented dangerous slip-and-fall hazards; the combination of wet feet and slick surfaces always seemed like a broken hip waiting to happen. Happily, today's trends are more spa-inspired and generally health enhancing. But of course there are exceptions.

LAYOUTS AND KEY FEATURES

One popular design trend with potential wellness downsides for two people sharing a master suite is the bathroom without a door. It can work if both individuals share the same work schedule, go to bed and wake up together even on their days off, and are both heavy sleepers. If not, the light and noise from one person using the bathroom can interrupt the sleep of the other.

Interrupted sleep can make someone sluggish, irritable, less mentally sharp, and more prone to a variety of illnesses. It also hinders muscle repair, which in turn hinders athletic performance. A healthier home for two has a door between the master bedroom and master bath. If you crave the open feeling and connection between bedroom and bath, consider a barn door with quiet glides.

Another trend that doesn't necessarily support well-being is the freestanding "trophy" tub. This stylish fixture is often positioned as the room's focal point, with only a floor-mounted faucet standing close to it. While a deep freestanding tub looks great, it can be difficult to get into and out of for some users—imagine trying this after an ultramarathon when your muscles are screaming at you already—and there's usually nothing to safely hold on to while doing so. Your only option is awkwardly bending to grip the rim while lifting your leg over it. This can be a particular risk to someone with balance issues, which many older adults have. A better option for safety is a built-in tub with a wide deck that you can sit on while getting in and out. It's not the trendy option but a much better one for those who love soaking.

On the other hand, the trend toward more spacious master bathrooms can benefit homeowners of all ages and abilities with improved accessibility to all of the fixtures. More floor space can mean easier use of the vanity, toilet, and shower. Larger stand-alone showers in place of tub-shower combinations are also a great convenience.

Another popular feature that can bring wellness benefits is the wall-hung vanity. In many cases, these stylish cabinets allow someone to roll under them if they're temporarily or permanently wheelchair-bound. They can also be installed at the height most comfortable for you.

These may seem like "nice to have" features now, but a serious injury can befall anyone (especially those engaged in adventure sports), and then "nice to have" becomes "must have," if only on a temporary basis.

Vanity areas can also be customized with modular storage to make getting ready for your day faster and more convenient. This might include organizers with electrical power in your base cabinet to hold your hair dryer or curling iron; a built-in refrigerated drawer for medications; LED lighting; a smartphone charger and speakers; and tall storage for linens and hampers. Having everything organized supports less stressful mornings.

HEALTHY BATHROOM COMPONENTS

One of the most desirable features of a master bathroom is a spa-inspired shower. In most cases it will have a bench, more than one type of showerhead, and a low- or zero-threshold entry, allowing you to walk (or roll) in without having to step over a raised lip. Such a shower can be a terrific health booster for the serious fitness enthusiast, especially with certain enhancements:

- A handheld showerhead with a massage setting will let you aim a pulsating jet of warm water at a targeted muscle group, much as sitting in a jetted tub would. It will also let you shower while seated if you're fatigued or injured, and clean grit, sand, or mud from hard-to-reach body parts for trail runners, hikers, and endurance athletes.

- A linear drain, which is a sleek, straight alternative to a standard centered round model, can be installed below a shower bench or next to a wall, which largely eliminates a trip hazard. This is especially true of the tiled-in versions, which minimize gaps in the tile that can catch a toe or cane, and those that mount directly on the wall where it meets the floor.

- A bench can serve as a comfortable perch for a standard or a steam shower, which brings benefits of its own. If you're in a rental, you can look for a stylish freestanding shower seat to serve the same purpose. Attractive models can be found online or at bath stores. Many are teak, which requires maintenance to keep its ruddy tones. A stainless steel model is a more maintenance-free option, but it will feel colder at first and can get uncomfortably hot, depending on your preferred water temperature.

- A steam shower can ease chest congestion, coughs, and allergies. It can also increase circulation and decrease blood pressure, reduce muscle and joint soreness, and open your pores.

There are cautions to using steam showers, though, including not staying in to the point of dehydration and making sure they're cleaned well so you don't catch another user's germs. (Low-maintenance shower walls, such as porcelain slab, will greatly facilitate cleaning.)

Do consult with your doctor before installing or using a steam shower to make sure it won't present any risks to your health. Your

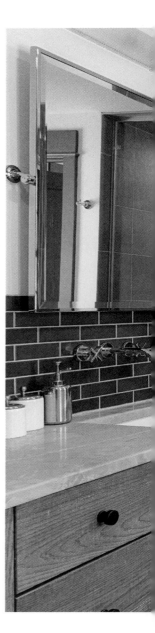

A linear wall drain eliminates a shower-space tripping hazard.

steam shower experience will also be enhanced with water filtration, so that you're not breathing whatever impurities and minerals are present in your well or local reservoir.

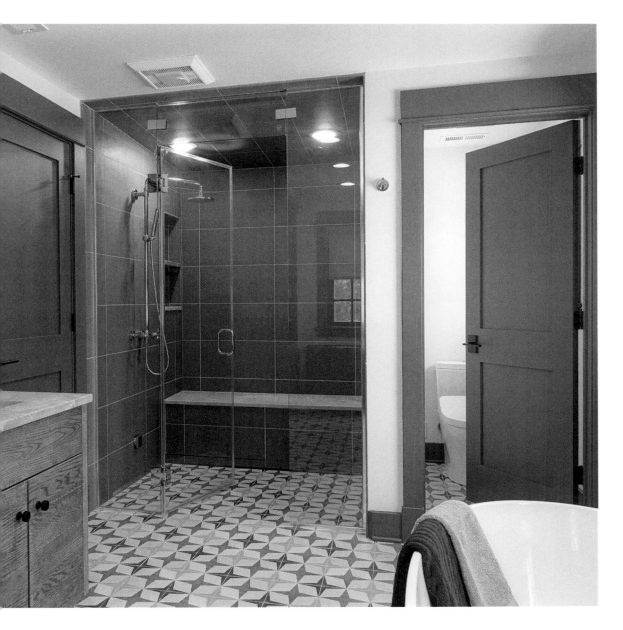

Bidet-style toilets are another health-enhancing bathroom component. They combine the features of a standard toilet with the intimate cleaning features of a bidet. Bidets are fairly common in Europe and Asia and are catching on in the United States, too, but as toilet add-ons rather than separate fixtures.

The benefits of personal cleaning with water rather than paper are less intimate irritation and potentially more thoroughness. Drying by warm air is also more comfortable than paper. This reduced discomfort is a boon to anyone who just spent hours in athletic shorts or on a saddle.

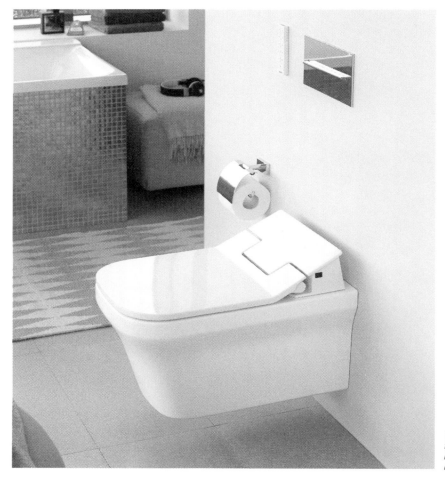

Wall-mounted, bidet-style toilets make personal hygiene and bathroom maintenance easier.

You can replace a standard showerhead in your owned home or rental with a handheld massaging version very easily, and take it with you when you move.

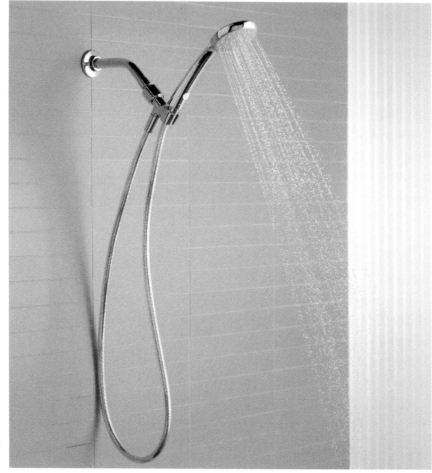

A handheld massaging showerhead can help ease muscle soreness after a tough workout.

It's fairly easy to install a bidet-style toilet in a standard bath-room remodel, as it fits in the same space as a traditional model. You'll just need to add electrical power nearby, which a licensed general contractor or electrician can provide.

If you're not remodeling your bathroom but want to enjoy a bidet's hygienic benefits, there are bidet seats you can add to many standard toilets. As with a bidet-style toilet, you will need to add electrical power close by to make the models with heated jets and dryers work.

Another toilet type to consider is the wall-hung model. This will allow you to adjust its mounting height to the user. A wall-hung toilet is also easier to clean. There are wall-hung models with bidet functionality as well.

One additional bathroom component with wellness benefits is plant life. Plants add tranquility and reduce stress reduction—they are ideal for a relaxing spa bathroom environment—and they can improve air quality. For bathroom spaces, choose varieties that love moisture and will thrive in your bathroom's light level. Your local gardening professional or a horticulturalist can help you choose the right plants for your space.

SAFETY WITH STYLE

Nobody wants to think about aging, injury, or illness, but we all get older and many times find ourselves dealing with temporary or long-term mobility challenges. A dual benefit of grab bars is to make our weaker moments—whether they be the result of a sports injury, a car accident, or just the adding of decades to our lives—easier and safer.

If you're remodeling your master bath, you can plan for future needs with structural blocking behind the walls. This means providing secure backers behind the walls so that weight-bearing bars can be installed at a later time. Or you can install grab bars during the remodeling process.

Just about everyone wants their master bath to look more like a resort spa than a rehab hospital room, so you'll be happy to know that new grab bar styles can be coordinated with the styles and finishes you choose for your faucets and accessories. Some incorporate towel bars or shelves so they don't even look like safety devices and blend into the space like any other feature. If you're not remodeling but find you need one or more of these safety essentials—or you just want to make getting into and out of a tub easier for yourself or a partner—look for models with specialized anchors for this purpose that don't require blocking, and be sure to install them (or have them professionally installed) according to the manufacturer's instructions.

In addition to making it safer and easier to get into and out of a tub, well-placed grab bars can make it easier to stand up from the toilet—no small feat after a twenty-four-hour endurance event or trail ultra!

HEALTHIER BATHROOM SYSTEMS

Your master bath should have the basic systems required of all modern buildings, but there is certainly room for improvement in many of them. These can add to your safety, comfort, and health.

A good ventilation system is an important starting point. A system not sized properly for a bathroom will not meet its needs. Nor will a vent fan that isn't properly installed. A noisy fan may be used less often—or not at all—and regular nonuse can lead to mold issues, which can be extremely unhealthy. A low-sone (meaning quieter) humidity-sensing vent fan designed for your room's size can help keep your bathroom healthier and more pleasant to use. You won't even need to remember to turn it on: It will sense when humidity has built up in the room and quietly turn on by itself. (This can be a definite advantage for vacation homes that are sometimes unoccupied.)

The quality of the bathroom's water is another health issue. We use it to brush our teeth, take our medicines, wash our faces, and clean our bodies. While the water we drink in the kitchen is often filtered at our refrigerator's dispenser or at the sink, many bathrooms lack filtration. This is a notable deficiency.

There are a few off-the-shelf filters that can attach to showers and bathroom faucets, but they're typically not attractive enough to fit the style of a spa-inspired master bath. If you're renting your place, these are worth considering for your well-being and can be taken with you or given away when you move.

If you own your home, the master bathroom is such a key feature when you sell, a whole-house water filtration system is really your best option. It will enhance the entire household's drinking, cooking, bathroom, and laundry water. As noted above, it will also enhance your steam shower if you have one.

Lighting is another system you may not think much about, other than the style of the light fixtures themselves. Updated building codes in many states mandate the use of energy-efficient lighting, which can mean fluorescent or, more likely, LED fixtures in your home. There are potential health issues associated with fluorescent lighting, largely due to its tendency to flicker and its color temperature (which affect how your eye and brain react to their light), and there are safety issues from the mercury inside if they're broken.

Fluorescent bulbs and tubes should always be handled with care and recycled. In many cases a fluorescent bulb in a light fixture can be replaced with an LED version. Check with the manufacturer or a trusted electrician before making the switch.

LED bulbs and fixtures should also be handled carefully if they break, as they, too, contain toxic elements. The good news is they tend to be very long-lasting, which means that you probably won't have to handle them for many years after installation.

More good news is that LEDs are now available in different, warmer-color temperatures, and are floor-illuminating and motion-activated or dimmable for that midnight trip to the bathroom. They also come in different formats for wall and ceiling light fixtures, night-lights, accent lights, and cabinet interiors. LEDs are even being built into showerheads, steam generators, spa tubs, and vanity mirrors for color-changing lighting in those areas.

Some people enjoy varying hues, especially when steaming or soaking, for mood and relaxation. This is called chromatherapy, and like other non-Western practices (e.g., acupuncture, aromatherapy, and reflexology) it may be beneficial to health. At the very least, it can create a relaxing mood for a bath.

LEDs have gotten considerably more affordable, making a

four-bulb fixture that gives you more illumination for putting in your contact lenses or shaving less expensive than an earlier three-bulb model.

There is some discussion among health professionals about LED risks, but they largely apply to the intense versions lighting city streets, not the more standard models used in the home.

LOW-MAINTENANCE BATHROOM MATERIALS

Cleaning the bathroom is probably no one's favorite chore, especially during sunny weekend hours when you'd rather be outside. So choose low-maintenance materials that make cleanup faster and easier. There are options today for just about every element of your bathroom, some with germ-inhibiting features.

Starting with your floor and walls, choosing tile with fewer and thinner grout lines will attract less mildew and be much easier to clean. Large-format porcelain slabs are an excellent option for bathroom wall surfaces. (Shower floors typically need smaller tile or nonslip surfaces for better traction.)

There are thin slabs large enough to cover many shower and toilet room walls completely. There are also larger, rectified floor tiles with grout lines as tight as an eighth of an inch. ("Rectified" means the edges have been engineered to be precise and consistent for closer installation and a more even surface.) If you're remodeling your bath-room, choose floor tiles with slip resistance. These are measured in coefficient of friction (COF) or dynamic coefficient of friction (DCOF), the newer standard, as discussed in chapter 3, "Material Choices." The higher the number, the less slippery the surface.

Toilets have traditionally been a gross nuisance to clean, but there are several worthwhile advances in this category that make them easier and healthier to live with. One feature is self-cleaning technol-ogy. This includes bacteria-killing light under the lid, interior mecha-nisms that do the cleaning for you, and cling-free bowl surfaces.

The cleaning you need to do on the toilet's exterior gets easier, too, with a full skirt or wall mounting. Both eliminate hard-to-reach and hard-to-clean spots on the outside. Some manufacturers have also removed handles in favor of hands-free flushing. This means less germ spread between users, which could result in fewer colds and flus bouncing around the household.

Look for low-maintenance benefits in your other bathroom choices as well, including cabinetry. The more decorative detailing your vanities have, the more time you'll spend dusting and scrubbing residue off of them. The glossier the surface, the more time you'll spend wiping off fingerprints. Matte-finish hardware and cabinet fronts will typically be easier to keep looking sharp than smooth, glossy versions.

Countertops are another area where you can reduce germs and cleaning time. A nonporous material, like engineered stone (also known as quartz) or solid surface (most popularly known by the brand name Corian), is an excellent option. Newer material offerings like porcelain slab are also low-maintenance and durable, and can be used for countertops or shower walls. These and more are also discussed in chapter 3, "Material Choices."

LUXURIOUS ADD-ONS

These are wellness enhancers worth considering if you're expanding the size of your master bathroom or building a master suite addition onto your home. It's not certain that they will significantly increase your home's resale value—you can check with a local real estate professional—but they can all contribute to your health and happiness while you live there.

- An outdoor shower extension brings the benefits of fresh air, indoor/outdoor living, and plant life to your master suite.

- Radiant flooring, which can be installed in a single room during a remodel or throughout a new-construction home, as mentioned previously, is delicious underfoot in a master bathroom on a chilly night or morning. (Some smart home systems include a geofencing app that turns the heat on or off when you come home or go out.)

- A towel warmer is a sensual luxury that can be installed by a licensed professional in a new or existing bathroom.

- An infotainment system can add relaxation to your bath with music, plus bring news, weather, and traffic updates to your morning routine while you get ready for work. It can also include chargers and holders to keep your electronics powered and safely stored while you're in the bathroom.

- Automated shades are ideal for hard-to-reach windows, like those above bathtubs, and add privacy and convenience to your master bathroom.

- Digital showering can automate each user's preferences in water delivery mode and temperature. There are even app-driven models that let you start your shower from another room and pause the water flow when it reaches your preselected temperature.

- Chromatherapy lights built into showerheads, steam showers, and jetted tubs add relaxation features to your master bathroom.

- A sauna is a big splurge with big benefits. Like steam showers, saunas have health benefits, but they use dry heat instead of moist. Like steam showers, they should also be used in moderation and only after consulting with your physician.

- Another big splurge is a flotation tub, especially one with zero-gravity features. Commercial spas with these tubs or tanks are gaining popularity; having one in your own master bath is a luxury. The one you visit at a spa may have salt water and sensory deprivation features, whereas your home model will use your own water supply and master bath environment. The flotation features—especially models with zero gravity—are designed to add a weightless feeling for extra relaxation. Combined with calming lighting and spa-inspired design, you can create an immersive experience that lets you unwind from a stressful day, with or without zero gravity.

- A fireplace can keep you warm when you get out of the tub or shower, and add relaxation and ambience to your bathroom. Be sure to consult with a fireplace professional in order to choose a clean-burning model that meets code in your area.

HOUSE CALL

The difference between steam and sauna is moisture. I may recommend one or the other, depending on what health condition I am treating. For respiratory distress from bronchitis or pneumonia, for example, steam can be helpful in breaking up mucus. I like to add eucalyptus oil for added benefit. A hot sauna is better for detoxification. Sweating out toxins—potentially from having to spend an evening in a smoky environment or overindulging in unhealthy foods or alcohol—is more effective in the dry heat, as it causes you to sweat more.
—Kristine Blanche, RPA-C, PhD, physician's assistant, Northport, New York; kristineblanche.com

A flotation tub is a serious wellness splurge for your master suite.

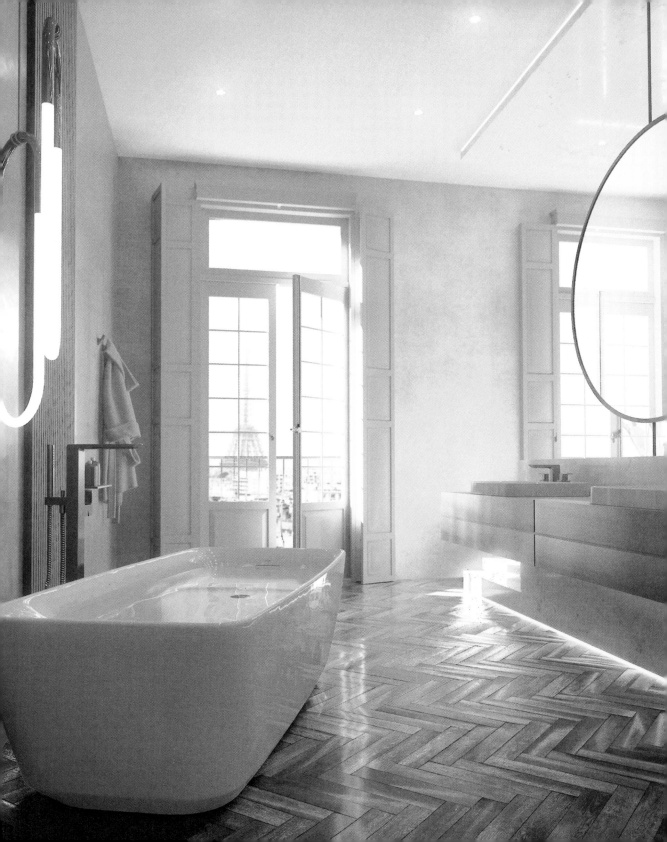

KIDS' BEDROOMS

Some of life's sweetest moments take place in your child's bedroom. That's where you tuck him in, where she writes in her diary, where you hug him after a heartbreak, where she gazes at posters of her favorite sports or entertainment stars. To a child or teen, the bedroom is his personal space for self-expression, homework, relaxation, and dreaming. It's where you let your kid be herself. At the same time, you need your child's bedroom to be a safe space that is conducive to the copious sleep all kids need. How do you create this?

NURSERY

The first room you'll likely create for your child is a nursery. This is where your baby will first experience color, shapes, movement, and life in your home.

In past generations, nurseries were often stereotyped into blue for boys and pink for girls, or a nongendered color like yellow for those who chose not to know their baby's sex in advance.

There are many more choices in favor today, and none is universally right or wrong. You can opt for soft greens that evoke open fields,

169

pale blues that echo clear skies, light grays that recall clouds, or soothing teals that whisper of Caribbean waves. The color is less important than the quality of paint in which it's rendered. This is one room in which you definitely want paints that don't off-gas.

The same is true for the furnishings of the room, from the flooring, crib, mattress, bedding, and changing table to the chair in which you'll rock your baby to sleep. All should be certified for indoor air quality. If your budget is limited, consider vintage pieces that you know are made of solid wood, not unknown composites, and hand-me-downs from eco-conscious family members and friends. (You can then pass them on to others or use with your second child.)

HOUSE CALL

Off-gassing from dangerous chemicals can cause damage in infant and child development. What we breathe is as important as what we eat. Toxins from flooring, paint, glues and other household pollutants can cause destruction to both adults and children. They are especially hazardous to youngsters, though, as their smaller bodies are still developing. Given how many hours babies and children spend in their bedrooms playing, studying, and sleeping, the potential amount of exposure they have to toxins can be dangerously high.
—*Maggie Berghoff, MSN, FNP-C, family nurse practitioner and functional medicine specialist, Nashville, Tennessee; maggieberghoff.com*

Carpeting tends to trap dirt and allergens and may off-gas into the room, making it a debatable choice for a nursery. Wool won't off-gas but it is a very expensive choice. If you're going to stay in the home for years, it could be a worthwhile investment. Wool is also available in carpet tiles if you're concerned about damage as your child grows or pets are allowed into the room. Nontoxic carpet tiles are another option for the same reason, potentially at a lower cost.

From a safety standpoint, you don't want to place the crib near a window or within reach of a window covering with a dangling cord, or have baby products in reach of the changing table. You also want that table to have a padded rug underneath and to buckle its safety strap around the child when you're using it.

Once your baby can get up on his knees or fully stand, you want to remove any hanging items above the crib. When she's able to crawl or walk, be sure all outlets are covered, extension cords are shifted behind furniture, gates and windows are secured so the child can't wander out, and furniture is fastened to the wall so it can't tip over. If you have a toy chest, make certain it has ventilation and a lid that won't slam down, catching a small hand or trapping your child inside.

Your nursery should have a working smoke detector and, ideally, an air purifier. If there's no carbon monoxide detector outside your baby's room, be sure to add one. There's medical research showing that using a ceiling fan in the nursery can reduce the chance of sudden infant death syndrome (SIDS),[1] making that a valuable addition to your baby's space. The theory is that the cool air circulating improves the quality of the air she breathes.

PERSONAL EXPRESSION

From an early age, children are able to express their preferences for colors and themes. This provides opportunities to create emotional wellness in their bedrooms. You can do it easily and affordably with decorative pillows, nontoxic accent rugs and no-VOC paints, which can be changed as your child grows and his tastes change.

If two or more children share a bedroom, you can give each one age-appropriate decorative accents in his or her favorite colors or themes, and combine the colors in window coverings or paint features. You can let your children help choose or create wall art that expresses their interests, possibly placing them in coordinating frames to emphasize family cohesion and elevate their significance over bare paper and tape. You definitely do not want to hang heavy or breakable frames over their beds, though, especially in a seismic zone!

BEDROOM ELECTRONICS

Many parents prefer to place the family's computers in an area where their use can be monitored, which can definitely be a safer alternative to having them in the kids' bedrooms. This also eliminates them as air quality and sleep disrupters. With phone and tablet proliferation at younger ages, it's getting harder to keep kids' bedrooms electronics-free. Given their blue-light screens, it's definitely worth the discipline, unless you can add automated filtering apps.

Blue-light issues with TVs—not to mention the off-gassing potential—can also be problematic in children's bedrooms. Removing these electronics from your kids' sleep spaces won't make you their best friend, for sure, but helping them get the hours of sleep they need means they'll do better in school and be safer on the road when they start driving.

LAYOUT

Layouts are definitely easier when there's only one child involved. Once two or more children share a room, it's important to consider their personal boundaries. Create separate spaces and storage areas for each child. He will appreciate not having his toys grabbed by a sibling and having his own relaxation zones to enjoy. Incorporate each child's personality into that zone via color, decorations, and furnishings so that it enhances his emotional health. Perhaps the younger will love a reading nook, while the older will prefer a hobby table. Sharing can be challenging but manageable if each child's space needs are addressed.

Many families opt for bunk beds to save floor space in a shared room. Pediatricians advise against top bunks for any child younger than six,[2] and frequently see injuries in children as old as ten.

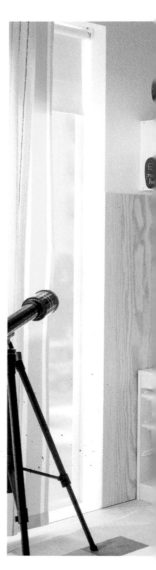

Bins and art for each child help create a healthy shared bedroom.

If bunk beds are a must, given room size restrictions, pediatricians also advise placing it in a corner so you can secure two of its sides, and ensuring that there's a guardrail on the top bunk. A soft, warm night-light will provide illumination so that the occupant of the top bunk can safely climb up and down the ladder.

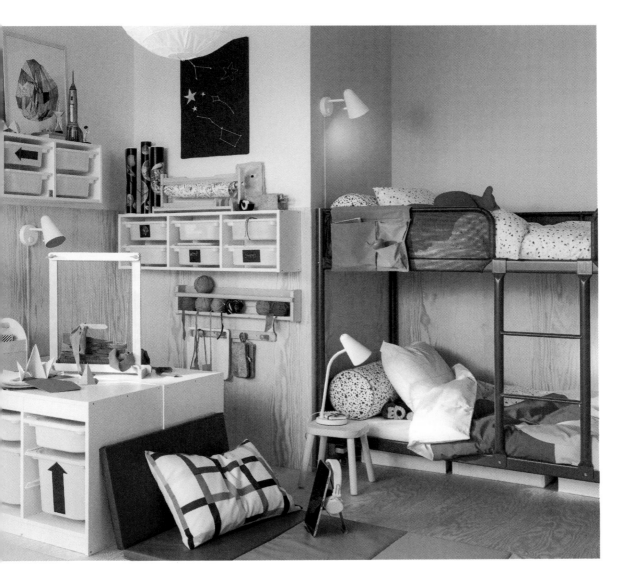

A trundle bed may be a safer albeit less convenient alternative. The challenge is for the child on the upper level to get out of bed without climbing over the child on the pull-out trundle. A model without a footboard—or a very low padded one—can help resolve that issue.

If the room's layout requires that more than one child share a desk, choose an adjustable desk light and desk chair so that each child's homework or study time can be well lit and comfortable. Give each an individual drawer or basket for supplies and a bin for papers. This will help ensure that homework and studying are more efficient and less stressful.

STORAGE

Parents often struggle to come up with toy storage solutions for their children's rooms. One option is to store most of their toys and games in their play area, if your home has one, rather than in their bedroom. Sleeping area space can be reserved for one or two small favorites that each child enjoys sleeping with. Overstimulation can keep children from falling asleep easily, and reducing the number of toys in their bedrooms also reduces the number of germs they're sleeping in close proximity to.

If your children's bedrooms are the only place to store their toys, select washable open bins that let them quickly see and reach their contents and just as easily return toys to them after play. If you have more than one child sharing a room, make each child's bin or bins his favorite color so that he knows which is his at a glance.

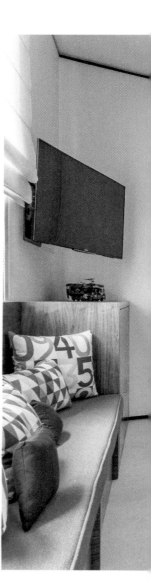

Built-in storage, an adjustable desk lamp and chair, and a blue-light setting on the TV can make this a healthy space a child can enjoy and grow with.

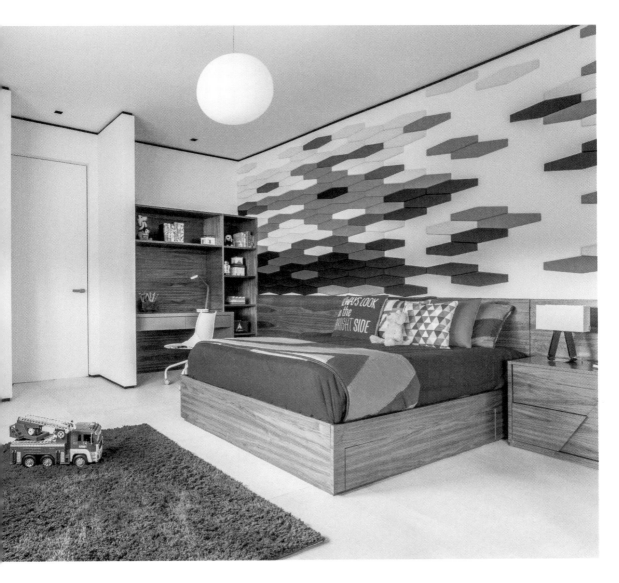

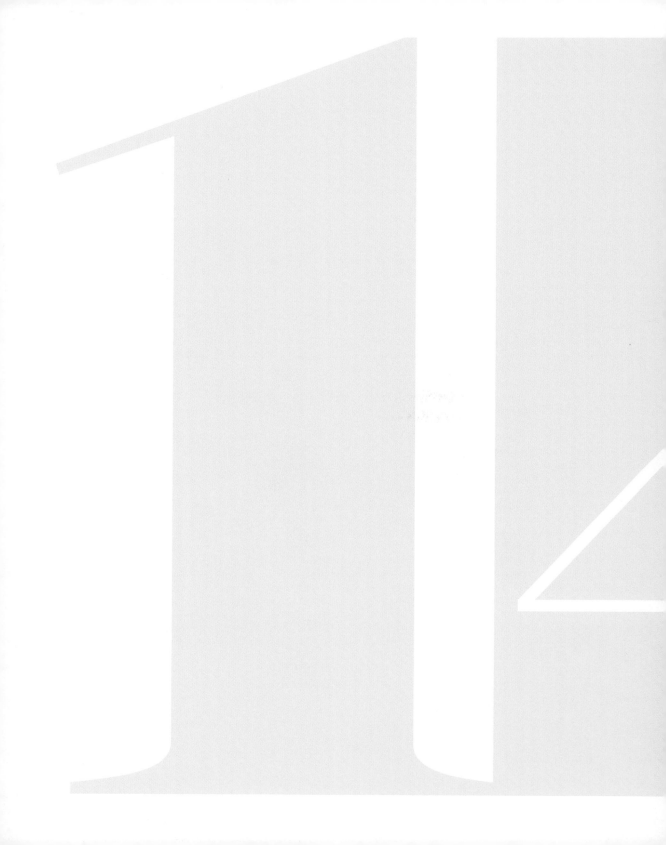

KIDS' BATHROOMS

Master suites get most of a home's bathroom budget, and powder rooms get most of its drama, but typically humble kids' bathrooms have an important role to play in their well-being and development. The bathroom is where they learn about hygiene at every stage of their lives, from toddler to teen.

In many single-family homes today, children have their own bathroom, separate from their parents'. It may be shared by more than one user and may just have one sink for multiple kids. There are two challenges with that setup: First, if more than one child is on the same school schedule, bathroom use must be coordinated carefully to get everyone out of the house on time. Second, cold and flu germs are spread more easily between family members by touching the same faucet.

There are some options to consider if you're redoing your kids' bathroom or building a home. One concept is the Jack and Jill bathroom, where there is a shared central tub and toilet room, with two separate vanity areas flanking it and connecting to separate bedrooms. This allows each child sink, vanity, and mirror use at the same time.

It also means each is touching only one faucet and vanity. If a Jack and Jill setup isn't possible, a bathroom with a double sink for two children is another option, as each still has separate faucet and storage space. If you don't have the space for two, a hands-free faucet is another option. You'll likely need to show your younger children how to use it once or twice, but once they're accustomed to doing so, it's going to save you cleaning time as well as reduce the spread of germs.

Two more germ spread reducers are touch-free light switches and a toilet with hands-free flushing. That's two fewer contact points for spreading colds and flu germs, and two fewer items you need to wipe down. (Yes, you'll have to show your kids how to use them at first, but young people are the original early adopters!)

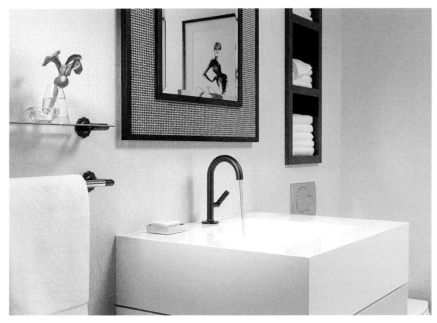

A hands-free faucet reduces the spread of germs in a shared bathroom.

While some homeowners opt for shower-only master bathrooms, kids' bathrooms almost universally get tubs. The tub in a kids' bathroom shouldn't be a soaking model, as its greater depth—often close to two feet—could require you to lift even older children to bathe them. A standard tub of less than eighteen inches is much easier to teach them to step in and out of as they grow.

There are some wellness opportunities to be had in the tub area too. One hazard that can be avoided with new technology is the tub set with a digital temperature display. This lets you bathe your young ones without you or them getting scalded or chilled. When the water reaches a comfortable temperature, you'll see it on the face plate or showerhead without having to test it on your skin or your children's.

HOUSE CALL

Scalding water can cause serious and painful burns that result in scarring, physical and emotional trauma, and possibly even the need for skin graft surgery. Remember to stay within reach of your child, particularly kids under six, while bathing to prevent burns or drowning. Keep young kids away from touching hot water faucets too.
—Dr. Jen Trachtenberg, MD, board-certified pediatrician, New York, New York; dr-jen.com

Another safety feature to consider for your children's bathtub is a grab bar. While these are mostly used for seniors, they add safety to active kids' bathing spaces, too, especially hand grips for when they're climbing in or out. You can find colorful, stylish models that will fit with the room's decor. Some can be installed in an existing bathroom without opening the walls for blocking.

When planning a bathroom update for young children who still need help in the tub, you'll find that a combination tub and shower with curtain and rod is more comfortable for your back than a bypass shower door. You won't have to lean over a metal track to wash them, and you won't wrench your back while reaching in when an active bather makes his way to the other side of the tub where a bypass door blocks easy access. A handheld showerhead will also be helpful to any parent assisting a child in the tub and cleaning it afterward.

Shower curtains have another benefit, especially when your child is at an age when she wants to express her own style, or if you have two children sharing a bathroom, each wanting a say in the room's décor. You can select a curtain with a color and theme that appeals to your children's sensibilities, associating hygiene with fun and creativity. You can do the same with coordinating towels, toothbrushes, cups, and bathmat. If your daughter's favorite color is red and your son's is blue, a red-and-blue-patterned shower curtain will please both, and each can have personal items in blue or red. (This will also reduce the spread of germs, as they won't have to wonder whose towel, cup, or toothbrush is whose.)

Whatever décor you add to your children's bathroom, you're going to want the space to be as clean and fresh as possible. A whole-house water filtration system will ensure that the water they use for washing themselves, brushing their teeth, and taking any vitamins or medicine is as pure as possible. A sensor vent fan will ensure that the air quality does the same. Children and teens often forget to turn fans on, so a sensor model will eliminate the memory factor and start operating when there's moisture in the air. This will keep mildew and mold away, creating a healthier bathroom environment.

One of the most common floor and tub surround materials for children's bathrooms is porcelain tile. It's a durable option with low-maintenance requirements when installed with minimal grout lines. If you're selecting new tile for a space you're updating, be sure to look for slip-resistant tile; wet feet and glossy surfaces can result in a painful fall. That may be less of a crisis than a grandparent falling, but it can still temporarily sideline a burgeoning dance or school sports career. Specialized treads or appliqués available in a home center or bath store can help reduce slips inside the tub if it doesn't have a non-slip bottom already.

If your children's bathroom has a window viewable from outside your home or apartment, you're going to want a privacy covering for it. If the window is in the tub enclosure, it will need to be water-resistant, of course. If you own the property, privacy film, a blind, or a curtain can work. If you're renting, a trimmed shower curtain secured with fasteners that won't damage the wall is an option.

WELLNESS FEATURE

Bidet-style toilets and seats are becoming popular for master bath use but can be a benefit in a child's bathroom as well. The water jets can improve hygiene between bath times and maybe even add a fun element to a child's experience learning about cleanliness.

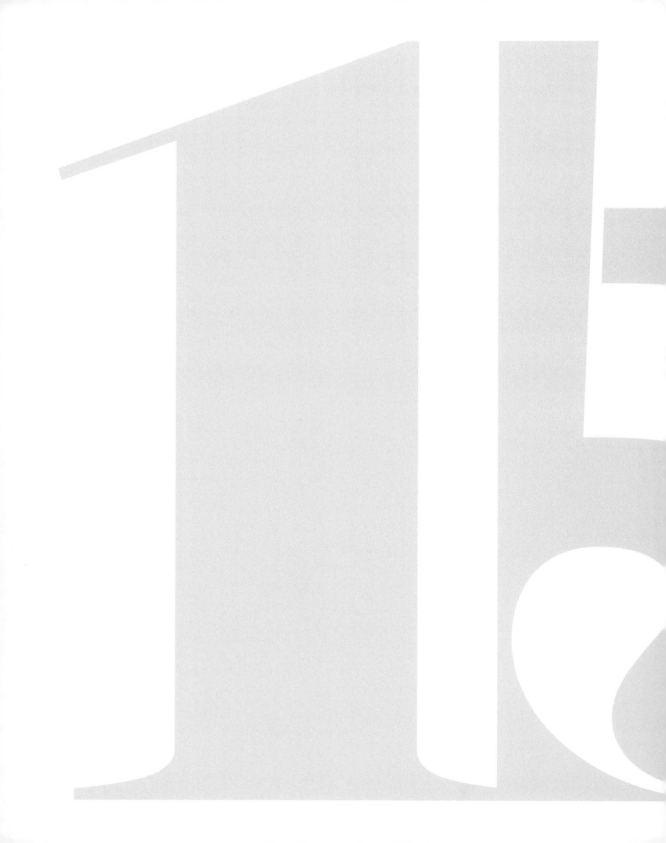

GUEST BEDROOM

Do you have a spare bedroom in your home where guests stay overnight? Some households have overseas family members who stay for weeks or months at a time. Others have running buddies who spend the night before an obstacle course race or marathon. Turning guest rooms into vacation rentals is also popular among people who live in desirable destinations.

GUEST ROOM CONSIDERATIONS

Think back to your own experiences staying overnight at friends' or family members' guest bedrooms when planning your own. Were they comfortable or cramped? Were they awkward spaces to use? Were they close to a full bathroom? What worked for you and what didn't?

Stay at least one night—ideally more—in your own guest room to see how it feels, and then see what can be improved for your guests to make it safe, functional, comfortable, and even enjoyable. Ask your guests for their honest opinion after they've stayed overnight and then follow up on their suggestions to enhance your space.

They may tell you that having a lamp on the nightstand would be helpful, so they can turn it off without having to navigate their way back to bed in a strange room in the dark. They may also mention that a bench at the end of the bed for holding their suitcases or putting on their socks would be helpful, as it would prevent someone with back issues or arthritis from struggling unnecessarily.

Many bedrooms are carpeted, and you may not be in a position to change it. The advantage of a carpet is its softness. Its disadvantage is its propensity to hide dust mites and other allergy triggers, as well as to potentially off-gas. Regular cleaning, especially just before guests'

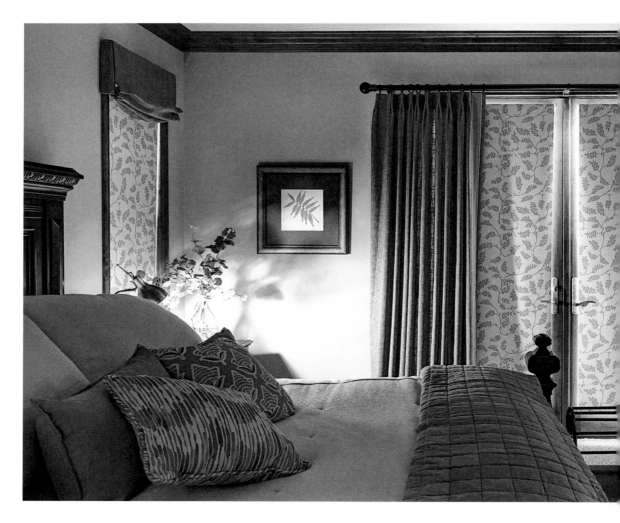

arrival, will help with the first. Air purifying systems and plants can help with the latter.

If you're planning a new guest room, you may want to consider either wool carpeting or wood flooring with a wool area rug (secured in place) for softness. (If you have a guest who is allergic to wool, it's typically triggered by skin contact, and socks or slippers should minimize the issue—unless they're going to meditate, pray, or do yoga on it.) A wool carpet or rug would not be suitable for a moisture-prone basement guest room, as wool is more susceptible to mildew and mold than synthetic carpeting.

ACCESSIBILITY

Are your guests likely to be seniors with mobility issues? In many households, especially those with relatives overseas, parents or grandparents spend extended periods visiting. Their mobility challenges should definitely be considered when planning a guest room.

There should be a clear, unobstructed pathway—ideally, wide enough for a wheelchair or walker—between the guest room door and the bed. A barn door is ideal to keep someone from blocking a door in a fall. (This applies to guest bathroom doors too.) If there isn't enough wall space for this option, consider a door that opens out into the hall, rather than one that opens into the room.

A nightstand with a lamp that can be turned on and off from the bed is important. There should also be room on top for a water glass, eyeglasses, and perhaps a book. Rounded front corners are helpful to reduce injury if someone with balance issues falls or bangs against it. The lamp and any ceiling fixtures should have sleep-friendly low- or non-blue bulbs, so as to not disrupt your guests' circadian rhythms. Blackout shades, liners, or panels are also great for achieving darkness.

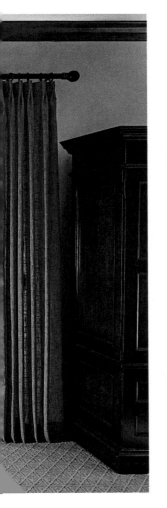

A bench, nightstand lamp, and blackout window coverings make a guest room more hospitable for overnight guests.

A circadian-friendly night-light (possibly motion-activated) between the guest bedroom and the bathroom that the guests will use can also add safety to their stay. You should also avoid situations where guests have to use stairs to transit between bedroom and bathroom. A first-floor guest suite is always ideal.

IN-LAW KITCHEN

If you regularly have long-stay guests, a kitchenette is also a valuable addition to a guest room. This turns it into what's often called an in-law suite. The kitchen features give both your visitors and your immediate family extra privacy. A mini-fridge, a convection toaster oven, a coffee maker, and a few place settings can make breakfast, snacks, and small meals possible. A compact dishwasher makes cleanup convenient. If your regular long-term guests have mobility or flexibility issues, a drawer dishwasher would be beneficial. You'll want handles rather than knobs for the cabinetry hardware, as they're easier to use for anyone with arthritis, hand tremors, or other grip-strength issues. Push-to-open doors and drawers without hardware are other good options. Make sure there's ample room in front of your kitchen area for a wheelchair or walker, so someone needing either can use the kitchen safely and easily.

BED AND BEDDING

Your guest may not have mentioned that she had a hard time sleeping because she was allergic to the down pillows and comforter on her bed. She might have thought it was just hay fever, but she sure wasn't feeling her best at the start line the next morning! Consider down-alternative pillows and bedding for guest rooms, and keep those clean and free of dust mites. Organic down alternative is even better!

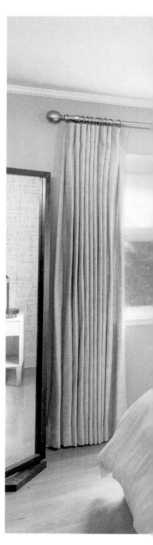

Treat your guests to organic bedding for healthier visits.

HOUSE CALL

People who experience allergic reactions to down comforters or pillows complain of eye irritation, respiratory and nasal symptoms, headaches, sleep disturbance, fatigue, and mood changes if the issue is not identified and resolved quickly.

—*Dr. Janette Hope, MD, FAAEM, DABEM, DABFM, diplomate of the American Board of Environmental Medicine, Santa Barbara, California; janettehopemd.com*

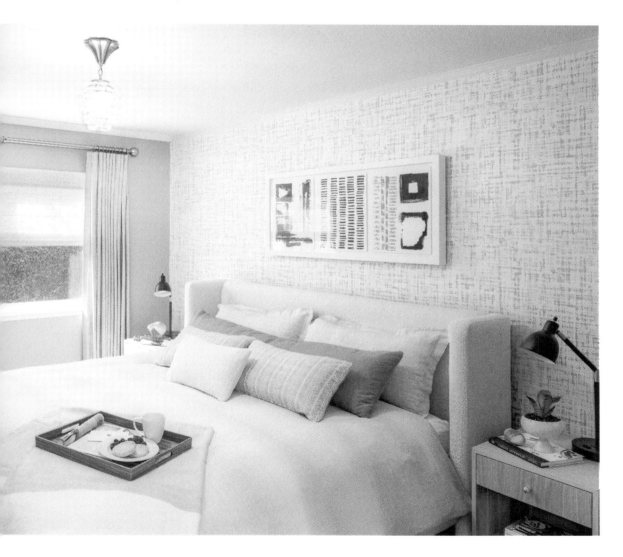

If you have regular long-stay guests, opt for a regular bed rather than a sleeper sofa. Most of those have thin mattresses and support bars that can make sleeping uncomfortable. (If your guest bed must double as seating, a daybed or convertible futon is often a more comfortable option.)

This isn't the room to house your ultra-high or ultra-low bed frame, either. You want to make it easy and safe for any guest to get into and out of bed, especially in the middle of the night.

CREATURE COMFORTS

Art, books, music, and hypoallergenic flowers like roses, daffodils, peonies, and tulips are nice touches for guest rooms. Plants are great for clearing the air, too, as long as you don't choose varieties that trigger allergies. Peace lilies, mother-in-law's tongue, and Chinese evergreen are good choices. Areca, lady, and bamboo palms are also good choices if you have room for a larger pot. (If your pets or your guest's pets are going to be sharing this space, know which plants and flowers are unhealthy for them; for example, peace lilies are harmful to cats and daffodils and tulips are harmful to dogs.)

Books about local attractions, such as where your guests can run, surf, hike, enjoy yoga outdoors, or get a massage, can be inspirational or informative. You may even have a pair of reading glasses handy on the nightstand. A yoga mat is a nice addition if there's enough floor space to use it.

Art can celebrate local attractions, local history, and culture or local artists. If you want to provide a creative outlet—which health professionals say can be therapeutic for those suffering from a range of physical and mental conditions[1]—you can include a sketchbook and colored pencils or markers for your guests to express themselves. A Bluetooth speaker can let them enjoy their favorite music with better sound quality than most tablets or smartphones offer while they read, relax, meditate, stretch, exercise, or sketch.

Slippers and robes are nice touches to make your guests feel pampered. Opt for organic fabrics if you can. Extra hangers in the closet, or hooks on the wall if closet space isn't available, will help your guests with their dressing needs. Be sure the smoke alarm is working in their bedroom, and that there's a carbon monoxide detector on the same floor. If the guest room is in your basement, add a radon detector as well. Your role as host is to make your guests comfortable, safe, and welcome.

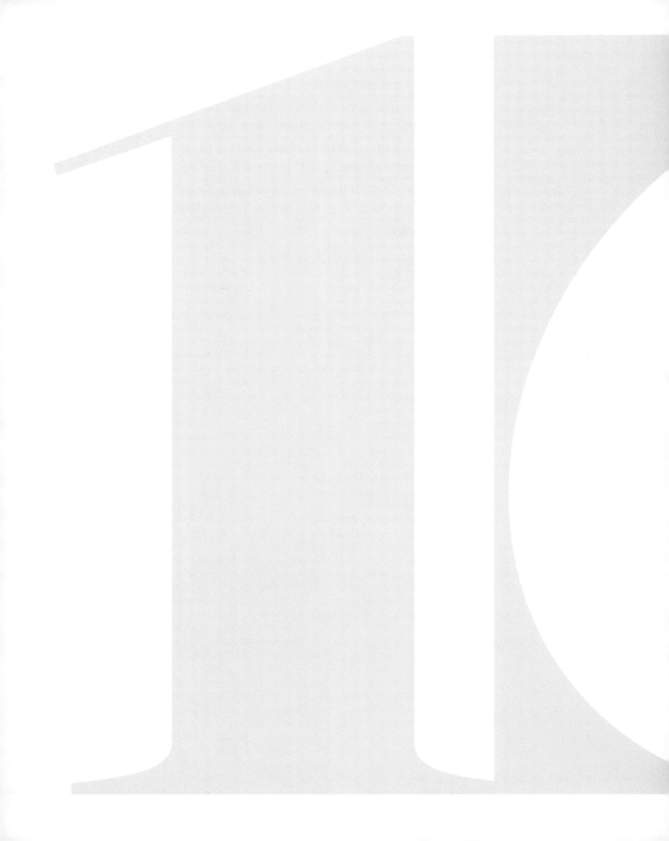

GUEST BATHROOM

Most modern master bedrooms have what are called "en suite" bathrooms—that is, the bathroom can be accessed directly (and usually exclusively) from the master bedroom. Increasingly, builders are creating town houses, condos, and single-family homes with more than one bedroom having an en suite bath. This is due to the popularity of multigenerational living, vacation rental hosting, and co-sharing arrangements.

Whatever the need, these private bedroom-bathroom pairings make great guest suites, as your visitors have the same level of privacy as their host. If your home has one, you're well positioned to have both short-term and long-term visitors.

How you'll equip your guest bath, regardless of its location, will depend on your typical visitor profile. Your long-term relatives will have different needs from those of your weekend trail buddy or your college roommate and his young kids who are staying for the week. Let's look at some universal principles, then at long- and short-term hosting needs.

ALL SPACES

If your home is older, you'll want to make sure you have an anti-scald shower set and valve. Earlier models without that protection have been phased out or mandated for replacement in most states, but older properties that haven't been sold in decades may have escaped updates. (If you ever had a shower suddenly go from comfortable to scorching when someone in another room flushed a toilet, it's likely that it had one of those non-upgraded fixtures.)

Since hot water can cause serious burns, especially in children, the elderly, or anyone unable to move quickly out of the way, you definitely want to be sure that all bathrooms in your home, including your guest bath, are equipped with anti-scald shower systems.

In a room where people will be showering or bathing, nonslip tile floors are generally the best option. They're durable, extremely water tolerant, and easy to maintain. Since they are very hard, though, a cushioned bath mat with a nonslip backing can cushion a fall if one happens. To reduce the chance of a guest suffering a fall while getting into or out of a tub/shower combination, opt for a standard-depth model and add a grab bar at its entrance.

It's also essential that every bath in your home, including those only used by visitors, has a functioning vent fan. This will help avoid mildew and mold buildup. That, in turn, makes cleanup easier and, more important, prevents mold-related illnesses.
A handheld showerhead makes it easier for your guests to clean themselves or their children and for you to clean up after them. If your regular guests are involved in athletics or have arthritis, a massage setting is a nice add-on.

A showerhead with push-button spray mode controls— as opposed to standard models that require the showerhead to be gripped and turned—is great for anyone with weak, shaking, or wet hands.

HOUSE CALL

Mold itself and its spores are not necessarily hazardous unless a person is sensitive or allergic to them. However, mycotoxins associated with mold spores can cause significant symptoms. When you inhale, touch, or ingest them, these natural poisons can lead to respiratory infections, chronic fatigue, kidney and liver disorders, Reye's syndrome and bone issues in children, and other conditions in people of all ages. Toxins of this kind can attack every organ and may lead to chronic health issues for a very long time afterward.
—*Dr. Carrie Lam, MD, DABFM, board-certified family medicine physician, Tustin, California; lamclinic.com*

LONG-TERM VISITORS

Someone staying for a month or more will have greater needs than someone coming for a day or weekend. If they visit every year—like parents traveling from overseas—this essentially becomes "their" bathroom, and it should be safe and functional for them. Consider push latches or handles, rather than knobs, for vanity drawers and doors. They're easier for anyone to open, regardless of grip strength or ailments. Lever handles on entry doors, faucets, the toilet, and the shower are also easier to operate.

If your long-term guests have mobility challenges—for example, if they use a walker or a wheelchair—you'll want to plan an accessible space so they can roll up to the sink, toilet, and shower easily. A wall-hung vanity and toilet make this easier. As mentioned earlier, a barn-style door or standard door that opens outward is also a good idea for guests with mobility issues; if they fall, they can't block the door from opening, and you can get to them faster.

A shower seat or bench and handheld showerhead on an adjustable bar will help users shower more safely. A grab bar near the shower entrance will provide safety when getting in and out. Another grab bar inside the bath or shower area will help while they're inside. There are many styles today that will blend in with the finishes and styles of your bathroom, so they won't detract from its aesthetic.

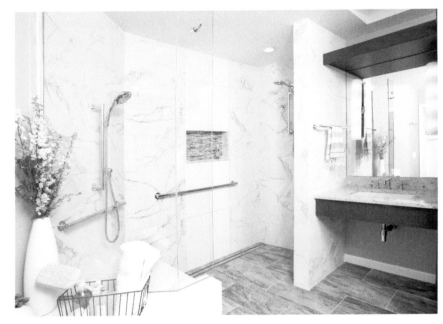

A bathroom with accessibility features adds value and "visitability" to your home for mobility-challenged guests.

Some cultures emphasize bathing over showering. If that's true for your guests, a grab bar for safer entry and exit from the tub will be especially important. You don't want someone grabbing a shower door or towel bar for balance. This is also a room where a standard-depth tub is going to work better for accessibility than a deeper soaking tub.

If your guests have vision limitations, creating contrast between the countertop, cabinet, and wall colors will make each surface easier to distinguish. Great lighting is also important for shaving, applying makeup, putting in contacts, and reading prescription bottle labels. Consider circadian systems that adjust for night use and better sleep.

SHORT-TERM VISITORS

If you're in a popular destination or have a large family or friendship circle, you may find yourself frequently hosting guests for a weekend or a week. They also deserve a safe, functional space but don't need as much storage or as many amenities as long-term visitors. Wall hooks to keep their travel bags off the counter will be helpful, especially if counter space is limited and you frequently have couples or families sharing a guest bathroom. Include coverings for privacy if the window can be peered into from outside.

A standard-depth tub that has a shower curtain and is easy to enter and exit and bathe children in will work for most guests. As with the shower, a grab bar near the entrance will make it safer to climb in and out. A quiet-functioning vent fan will do the job for most short-term guests.

If you often host family members with young children, hooks will make it easier for multiple bathroom users to hang their towels after use, and a step stool that can be moved out of the way when not needed will help the smallest visitors reach the sink. (A step stool with storage can also hold bath supplies in cramped rooms.)

Here's something to consider if you are a short-term rental host: If your home—including its guest bathroom—is accessible to guests with mobility challenges, you may find yourself booked more regularly, as accessibility isn't as common as it should be. There are also websites for these travelers that can give your property extra exposure.

HEALTHY PAMPERING

Sharing your home with friends, family, and even paying guests can be fun and rewarding. Consider having soaps and shampoo without dyes or perfumes, extra toothbrushes, and dental floss on hand. Organic cotton robes, slippers, and towels are a great touch. Radiant floor heating and towel warmers are next-level pampering that will make your guests feel truly relaxed and refreshed after a long day of hiking, cycling, or skiing.

LAUNDRY/FLEX ROOM

The house you grew up in might have had its washer and dryer in the basement or garage. Laundry rooms have grown in size, function, and style since they first started to emerge in suburban homes a couple of decades ago.

It's not uncommon to see a laundry/flex room (typically a customizable, multipurpose space) almost as large as a kitchen in a new-construction home, with attractive cabinetry and distinct "zones" for laundry, crafting, and even pet needs. This creates an appealing, low-maintenance space for chores and hobbies. When your laundry area is bright and cheerful, it makes the work so much less dreary! And when there's room for your hobbies, too, you'll have a pleasant place in which to enjoy your time more even while doing mundane housework.

If you're in an apartment or converted condo, you may share a laundry room full of machines with the rest of the building, although in-unit hookups are more common today than they've been in the past. Skip to the next chapter if you're not planning on buying a home with a laundry room soon and if you don't have one now.

SURFACING

Laundry/flex rooms are often tiled in the same material as your entry for easy-to-clean, water-tolerant sturdiness. Rectified porcelain with extremely tight grout joints will be an extremely low-maintenance, durable choice. If your laundry/flex room is going to get extra-hard usage, like regularly cleaning muddy pets, hiking boots, and backpacks, for example, you might also want to consider sealed concrete with cushioned anti-fatigue mats where you'll be standing for long periods of time.

Scrubbable no- or low-VOC paint is the most practical wall surfacing option for easy cleanup in these heavily used spaces. If the ceiling is low and splatter risk is high—by a wet dog, perhaps—consider painting the ceiling in a scrubbable paint as well.

LAUNDRY APPLIANCES

If your laundry area only has enough room for a washer and dryer, it won't serve well as a flex room, but you can still choose a laundry set that can enhance your wellness. Size factors in with that choice too.

If you can only fit a stacked pair, you're limited to stackable front loaders. There's nothing wrong with that choice, unless you happen to be short. That makes reading the controls on the stacked dryer more challenging. New Wi-Fi–connected appliances let you operate the controls from your phone, tablet, or smart speaker, making it unnecessary to climb up on a chair or stepladder to read the buttons or dials near the top of the dryer. That can be helpful.

If you have room for a side-by-side pair, you can opt for front or top loaders, depending on which feels more comfortable for you. Front loaders often require bending, which may not be easy on your back, especially with larger laundry loads. Pedestals that mount under the machines can put front loaders at a more ergonomic height but make folding clothes on top of them less comfortable. It's up to you to decide which serves you better, knowing that both options are available. If you have another place to fold, perhaps with a fold-down table on the wall, the pedestals can be a worthwhile investment.

Washers and dryers have numerous features today that older pairs lacked. For one, they're usually more energy- and water-conscious than older models. Look for the Energy Star label to ensure both, then use the savings on your utility bills to spend on more gear, an extra race, or a nutritious cooking class!

Some washers now offer steam settings, which help sanitize clothes, remove allergens, and fight odor and stains better. If your fitness activities involve dirt and mud, or you or a household member have allergies, a steam washer can be a health-enhancing choice for your home. On the flip side, it will cost more than a non-steam washer and may require a longer cycle.

Steam-equipped dryers also cost more than standard models but can save you ironing time. You can also use a steam cycle just to freshen a load of laundry without doing a full run. A fabric steamer can do the same job at a lower cost.

Whichever set you buy, be sure to maintain the machines according to the manufacturer's recommendations. This will protect this expensive equipment as well as your clothing, bedding, and towels.

There's a fairly new class of laundry appliance called a refresher. It's designed to remove odors and allergens from your clothing, towels, and bedding and even your children's stuffed animals, which can be beneficial to some households. It can also spruce up your suit before an important meeting, neaten your yoga togs in time for class, and take the smoke out of your favorite little black dress if you ended up on the wrong patio.

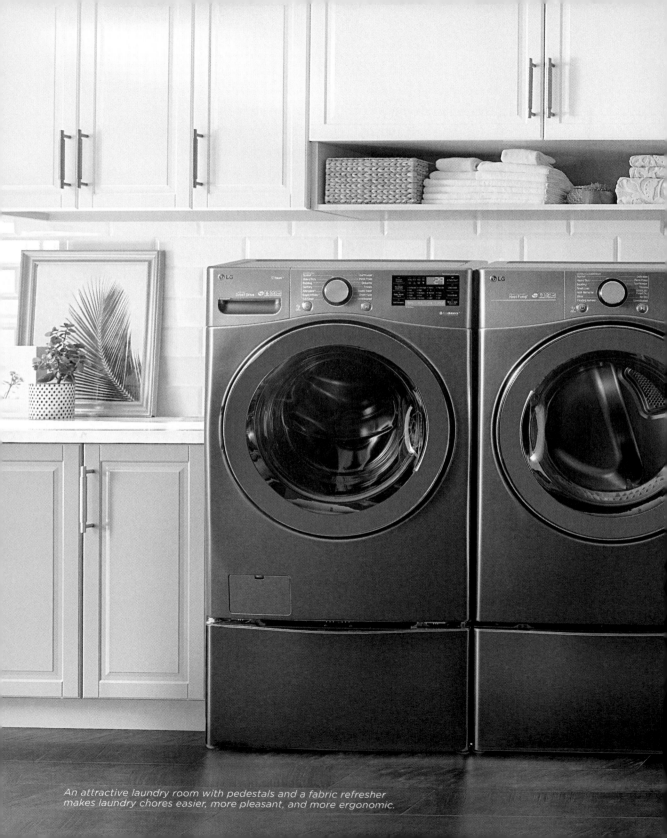

An attractive laundry room with pedestals and a fabric refresher makes laundry chores easier, more pleasant, and more ergonomic.

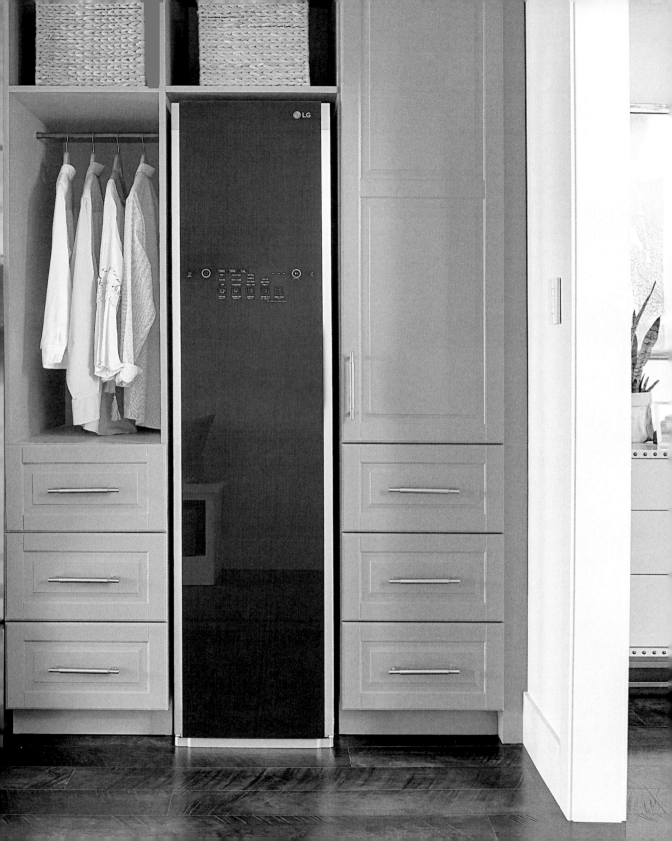

SINKS AND FAUCETS

If you have room for a sink, it's a fabulous fixture for cleaning items you wouldn't want to machine wash, like a wetsuit or trail shoes. Look for the largest, deepest model you can fit into the space you have available. Some models are floor or wall mounted. Others are intended to be installed in a cabinet and countertop; these tend to be more attractive but are often smaller. Restaurant supply stores can increase your sink selection over home centers or kitchen and bath showrooms.

A pull-out faucet will give you more functionality than a standard utility sink model when cleaning bulky items (or pets). Choose a model with lever handles and a low-sheen finish for easier handling and cleanup.

LAUNDRY/FLEX ROOM STORAGE

Where do you hang or lay your hand washables to dry? Planning this capacity into your laundry/flex room is ideal. A drying rack mounted high on a wall over the sink can hold your wetsuit after a triathlon or scuba trip and provide a space to hold a backpack and trail shoes while they're drying.

Having a single designated spot in your home for all of your athletic gear makes it faster and easier to grab what you need before heading out the door. Having the gear section of your home sharing space with your laundry facilities can make after-event cleanup and storage more convenient too. Your gear can go from washer, dryer, or refresher straight into designated storage for its next use. Some items, like wetsuits, need to be stored away from direct sunlight, so a laundry room wall away from a window can be ideal.

Your laundry area storage space can also include a cabinet or cart for supplies, a trash bin, and a hamper to hold clothes between washings. If you have creative or athletic hobbies, you might also plan storage for those, as the room's sink would be a great help in washing your hands and equipment after an art or gardening session.

Your flex space may have room for a table or countertop for folding laundry, doing chores, or enjoying your hobbies. These all work well in a laundry room with a sink, as it's perfect for cleaning yourself, your gear, and your work surface.

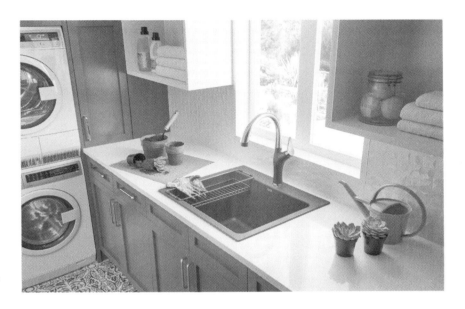

Laundry rooms can double as pleasant, functional "flex" spaces for healthy (and messy) hobbies like gardening.

Whether you mostly sit or stand while using your work surface will influence its height and seating needs. Kitchen counter height (thirty-six inches) works well for standing tasks. A counter stool with a back can provide comfortable seating on those occasions when you don't want to stand. Table height (thirty inches) is perfect for activities you'll spend longer hours completing while seated. Choose a comfortable, ergonomic rolling chair or stool with low-maintenance materials for this purpose.

PETS

If you have pets, consider adding storage for their needs in this utilitarian room. Flex rooms are also great for setting up pet feeding stations and sleeping space. A low-maintenance floor will handle any food spills until you can deal with them, and they won't be eating in your kitchen, underfoot, while you're cooking or cleaning up. That's safer for both them and you. (Tripping on pets is a sadly common hazard for the elderly.)

Larger laundry/flex rooms are becoming popular spots for dog-washing stations. Adding one is similar in cost and complexity to adding a shower to your own bathroom, minus the spa add-ons like steam or a rain showerhead. Think of it as a kinder, gentler option than a hosing down on cold days for your favorite running or hiking buddy. Elevating a pet shower to make it kinder on your back is an option if a larger dog can still get in and out on its own, or if your pet is small enough to safely lift. A handheld showerhead makes cleaning the pet and the space afterward much easier.

Pet features like dog showers, beds, and feeding stations offer wellness benefits for you and your four-legged friends.

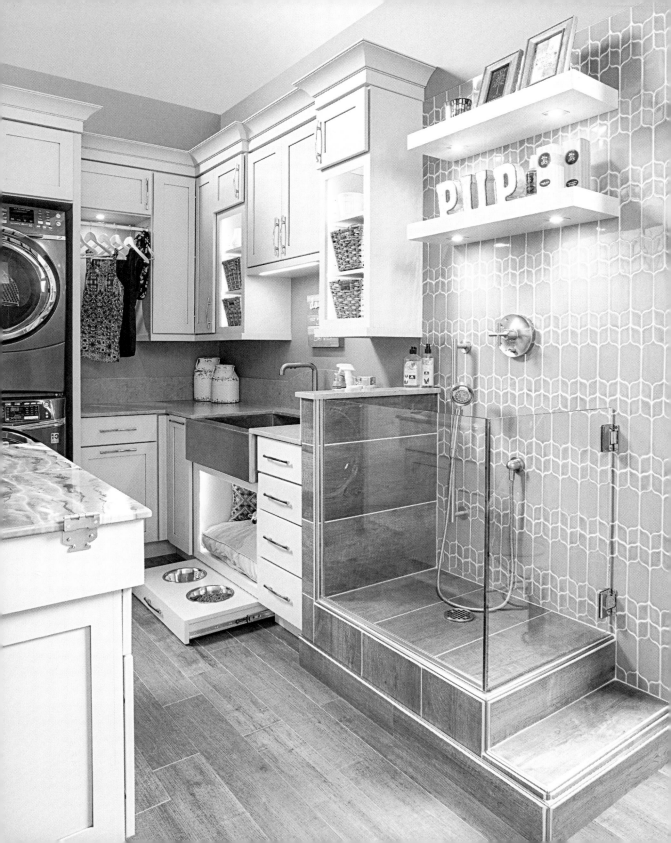

LIGHTING

It's great when laundry rooms have natural light coming in from windows, solar tubes, or skylights, but they don't always, especially if they're in your basement. Be sure to include both ambient and task lighting if you have more than a laundry closet. The ambient lighting will provide illumination for the entire room, while task lighting will focus on specific areas where you work or enjoy your hobbies.

Ceiling fixtures or recessed or track lighting can provide ambient light for the room, and dimmers are ideal for softening their glow. LEDs provide the most energy-efficient, long-lasting solutions.

Add lighting at the spots where you do the most work, like at the sink, over the washer and dryer, at the pet center, and above any table you add to the space. If you have wall cabinets or shelves above these surfaces, task lighting can be mounted to their undersides. The key detail is having enough light shining on your work area so that you can see what you need to see—whether it's the instructions on a garment label or watering instructions on a plant tag—without eyestrain.

DECORATION

Most people don't relish doing laundry, and having to do it in a dreary space makes a time-consuming, routine chore even less pleasant and something that saps a little bit of joy from your life every week or more.

If you brighten your laundry space with wall paint in your favorite cheerful color, a decorative anti-fatigue mat on the floor to reduce stress on your joints, and fun personalized artwork on the wall that makes you smile when you look at it, you can add a bit of joy to your laundry chore. It's amazing how much a fun visual can lift your mood on your least favorite part of your week. (Having a smart speaker for streaming your favorite tunes while loading laundry or cleaning gear helps too.)

WELLNESS TIP
Consider a vintage travel poster that transports your mind to your favorite vacation spot, or handsome photographs of the mountain you're planning to climb next season. Delight hor inspire yourself for a mental health enhancement.

Natural light, ergonomic folding space, and a pleasant setting make laundry a less tedious chore.

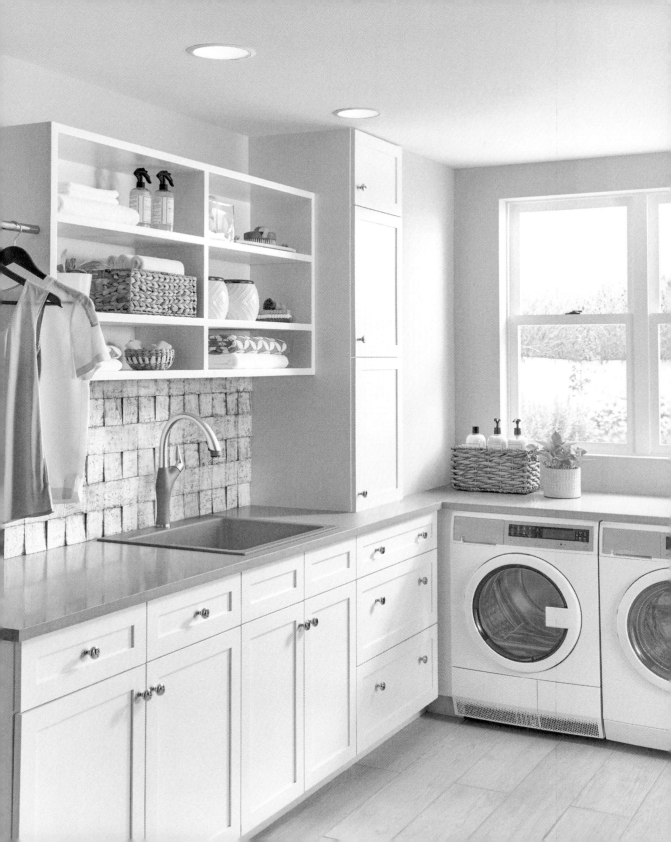

GARAGE

Garages have become parking spots for more than cars. People tend to park their bicycles and other sports gear there as well. What's in yours? Surfboards, wetsuits, hiking poles, tents, ice skates, golf clubs, backpacks, and skateboards often find themselves stored in a garage, sometimes in a heap, sometimes in organized "zones."

It's not uncommon to find other essentials stored in garages, too, sometimes for years. These can include gardening tools, paint and paint supplies, home repair tools, emergency kits, and old files. When was the last time you looked through the items taking up space in your garage? Some may need to be discarded or donated. Some may need to be safely handled and disposed of—especially old chemicals that shouldn't go into your local water system. Garage sorting is almost no one's favorite chore, but it can be helpful to your mental and physical health. It can also free up space for other, better uses.

It's not one of those "out of sight, out of mind" chores, either; every time you drive into your garage or return from a bike ride, you'll be facing the same clutter and undone task. That does not create a positive welcome-home mood.

SPACE PLANNING

If your garage could be cleared of expired supplies, gear you haven't used in the last decade, files you can digitize, and those donation bags you never got around to dropping off, what would you do with that freed-up space? Maybe you've been longing for a craft or workout room, but there's no space in your home, or maybe you've been eyeing a potting table for gardening. All of these can "live" successfully in a garage.

If you're active in a gear-intensive sport like surfing, kayaking, scuba, hiking and camping, or cycling, creating a zone for gear in your garage makes great sense. You'll want space for storing items in a way that protects them when they're not being used and makes it easy to access them when you're ready to head out the door.

The first step in your space-planning process is to determine how much room your gear requires, what type of storage—for example, shelves, hooks, or specialized racks—is required, and where in the garage you can accommodate both. You'll need to factor in room for your car and walking space around it. If your gear is going to need regular washing after use to keep it in good condition, can you plan your zone to include your garage's utility sink or hose connection?

Do you have space that you haven't considered before, like overhead or in an unused golf cart bay, since you sold your clubs a decade ago? Ceiling space can be leveraged for seasonal items to rotate in and out of and for items you're planning on giving away in the future.

An unused golf cart or car bay can be repurposed as a hobby space. Will you need an electrical outlet, if not for tools to repair or maintain gear, then for task lighting? Would a worktable or counter be helpful? If so, how large should it be and how high off the floor will be most useful and comfortable? Will you be standing or sitting while you use it? For how long? That will determine whether you need a counter stool, chair, or anti-fatigue mat to stand on for extended periods.

If you're going to be using your garage for more than storage, climate control will become important, especially if you're exercising

WELLNESS TIP
This might be a good opportunity to connect with a professional organizer in your area. At the very least, it sets a deadline for getting started with a difficult chore that might otherwise keep getting pushed back week after week.

A well-organized garage can host a well-equipped workout space.

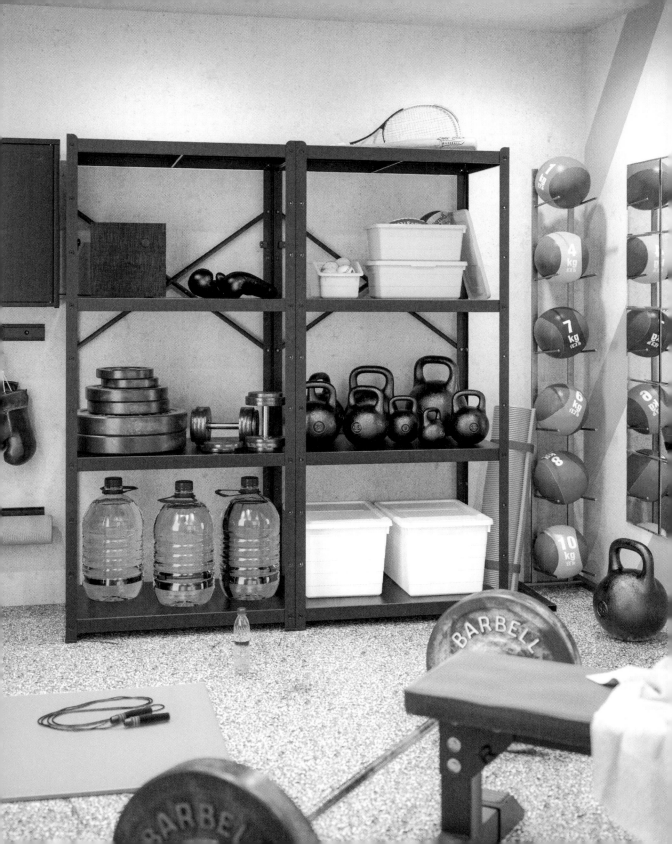

there in the hotter months. Garages aren't generally heated or cooled, so how will you spend time in that space comfortably? While central heating and air is generally not an option, space heaters and fans can certainly help. (Be sure to plug your space heater directly into an outlet, not an extension cord or surge protector!)

If your garage has a window, a window air-conditioning unit could be an option. These typically require electrical power, so plan your zone to include an existing outlet, or bring in a licensed electrician to add one where it will be most helpful. Outlets are rarely as abundant in garages are they are in homes.

If you're going to spend many long happy hours there, a ductless heating and air-conditioning system may be a good option. There are online calculators to properly size one of these energy-efficient systems for your garage. Whatever option you choose for your climate control and for any high-load electrical tools or appliances, be sure you have a safe and ample electrical supply available. A licensed electrician can be helpful in guiding you to your best code-compliant solutions.

If you are planning on working out in your garage, space planning is especially crucial. Treadmills and stair climbers need a power source, and all equipment has unique clearance needs so that you can safely get on, get off, use, park, and walk around it. Check the manual before you buy and bring something home. You'll also want a fan and a place to hold a water bottle or dispenser if the fitness equipment doesn't have a built-in holder, just as with indoor fitness spaces. (Note that it can be easier to dehydrate when working out in a hot, non-air-conditioned garage.)

It's good to answer all of these questions for yourself before creating a storage, hobby, or fitness zone in your garage. It will help you factor in size, features, and cost. Here are some of your options.

STORAGE

You may have hundreds or thousands of dollars invested in your sports gear, and properly storing it will protect that investment. Bikes, kayaks, and surfboards need quite a lot of space, and all can be weighty, but each has a different set of specialized holders.

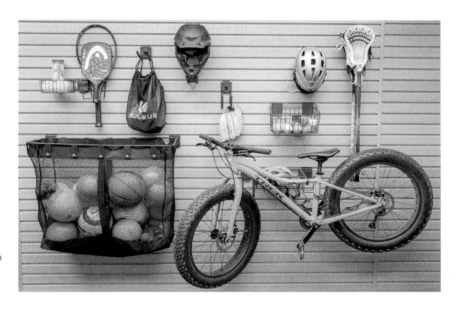

Having your sports gear safely stored and easy to reach means getting out the door faster and with less stress.

Where you install them will depend on your available room vis-à-vis your car, household storage, hot water tanks, and other items in the garage, but you should also consider your upper-body strength in lifting gear on and off wall- or ceiling-mounted holders. A kayak can weigh fifty pounds, something to keep in mind if you're planning on storing it overhead!

Wetsuits shouldn't be folded or stored near chemicals or in direct sunlight. They also don't like auto fumes, so a closed cabinet is best if yours will stay in the garage. Learn about the storage requirements for your sports equipment to keep it in peak condition for as long as possible.

Some sports gear is small and easily misplaced in a large garage. Bins to organize these items by sport—like hiking/trail running and scuba/snorkeling—can keep you organized and ready to go at a moment's notice. After cleaning, these items will always be returned to their specialized bins for storage. These bins can "live" on garage shelving in easy reach and close to the larger gear racks. Ideally you will be able to head out on a spontaneous or long-planned adventure with everything clean, accessible, and ready to go when you are.

Some sports, such as skiing and snowboarding, are seasonal, and your gear can stay in overhead garage storage for many months when not in use. It's good to have more accessible holders for busy seasons, though, so you don't have to constantly get things down from above when you want to use them. If you participate in summer and winter sports, as many people do, you can rotate gear from accessible to overhead long-term storage as the season demands.

If you're storing household chemicals in the garage—especially if you're also using the space for hobbies or exercising—it's essential to store them safely. You don't want them off-gassing into your workout space, and you don't want them leaking onto your sports gear. After making sure that they haven't expired, store them in a cabinet or bin that won't be damaged if they do leak.

HOUSE CALL

Flip around that spray paint, bug killer, weed treatment, and all of those other household chemicals you store in the garage. You'll likely find a list of toxins that are linked to cancers and endocrine disorders. It is extremely important to keep these items out of reach of children, and not to use them around children when possible. When you do need to work with these products, do so in a well-ventilated area with the windows open. You really don't want to be breathing these fumes or subjecting your family to them.
—Maggie Berghoff, MSN, FNP-C, family nurse practitioner and functional medicine specialist, Nashville, Tennessee; maggieberghoff.com

SECURITY

Is your garage secure? If it's in an apartment building and shared with other tenants, your space might include its own lockable cabinet for small items. That won't protect your bicycle, kayak, surfboard, or other large gear, though. Fortunately, there are locking racks you can use to secure these in a shared garage, or even in a single family or town house community where burglars or opportunity thieves frequently prowl. U-shaped locks are generally harder to break than cable locks, so consider those for securing your gear to its specialized racks.

Thieves often roam neighborhoods looking for open garage doors or unlocked service doors so they can get in, steal any visible items, and dash out. You can avoid being victimized by adding a dead bolt to your service door, covering its window if there is one and getting an automatic garage door opener with a timer or smartphone app that closes the door remotely. It's not uncommon to forget to close your garage door after unloading everything after a big trip; the automatic garage door opener will close it even if you forget, or you can direct it to do so via Wi-Fi. (If you're concerned about getting locked out, an exterior keypad can get you back in.)

Motion sensor lighting at your garage entrance will also deter thieves. One of a home's greatest vulnerabilities is its garage door. Knowledgeable thieves can access its emergency release cord with a push at the door's top section and a grabbing tool. You can buy or make your own cord block. If you're handy or have someone who helps you with tasks like these, you can add a lock to your garage door track to stop someone from backing a truck up to your home, opening the door, and loading all of your valuable gear into it while you're out of town. There are also inexpensive DIY motion-activated cameras with night vision that can alert you on your mobile device anytime there is something or someone within range of the front of the home.

STYLE

Do you usually come home by car? If you live in the country or sub-
urbs, you probably do more often than not. That means it's your garage
that welcomes you first in all of its utilitarian glory. Garages often have
gray concrete floors, bare walls, one basic ceiling light, and no decoration. Even without clutter, they're generally not warm, comforting
spaces. Why not add elements to your garage that will greet you with
more style? After all, this is the space that most of us traverse at least
twice a day, almost every day.

You can paint the wall with your home's entry door your favorite
accent color. You can hang a medal rack where you'll see it as soon as
you drive in. Runners can hang their race bibs along a wall, creating a
reminder of all of those great times. Mountaineers can add posters or
photographs of their favorite summits. Surfers, divers, and kayakers
can add pictures of their favorite waterways.

There are so many ways to welcome yourself home with a more
uplifting visual than "garage basic." By making the first view inside
your residence a smile-generating experience, you give yourself an
easy, instant mood booster each time you return.

If you're going to be spending hours in the garage with a hobby
or exercise equipment, it's even more essential to make it an attractive
space. You may have to set up a table with shelving, seating, a task light,
and a storage cabinet to participate in your favorite hobby. That will all
make it functional. Perhaps paint the table and cabinet a fun color that
coordinates with the chair or stool. Add complementary color to the
walls with paint and/or decorative elements. Include an outdoor-rated
rug for low-maintenance style, or an attractive anti-fatigue mat if you'll
be standing at the table for long hours. Select seating that's ergonomic
for the task you'll be performing there, just as you would for your home
office—especially if you'll be sitting for extended periods. Adjustability
in height and back angle is ideal.

Choose a task light that adds style as well as illumination. Add a beverage cooler or water dispenser to stay hydrated without having to run into and out of the kitchen.

GARAGE WORKOUTS

Group garage workouts have become more popular in recent years, especially with the growth of endurance sports and boot camps. These often emphasize camaraderie and body weight work over elaborate gear. You may have friends who have organized garage workouts at their homes. You may have done the same—or want to.

There are gigabytes of online workouts you can do in your garage with friends, some needing little more than kettlebells, jump ropes, and boxes. Adding rubber mats to your garage floor will increase comfort. So will adding a heavy-duty fan for workouts on hot days. If you're going to be hosting often or working out on your own regularly in your garage, having a water dispenser or mini-fridge with water or hydration drinks available in your gym zone can be helpful.

Last but definitely not least, if you're going to add a climbing rope or other elements that need to be permanently installed, make sure that you're using the right hardware and properly securing it to something with structural integrity that can handle the load. And update your homeowner's policy for peace of mind!

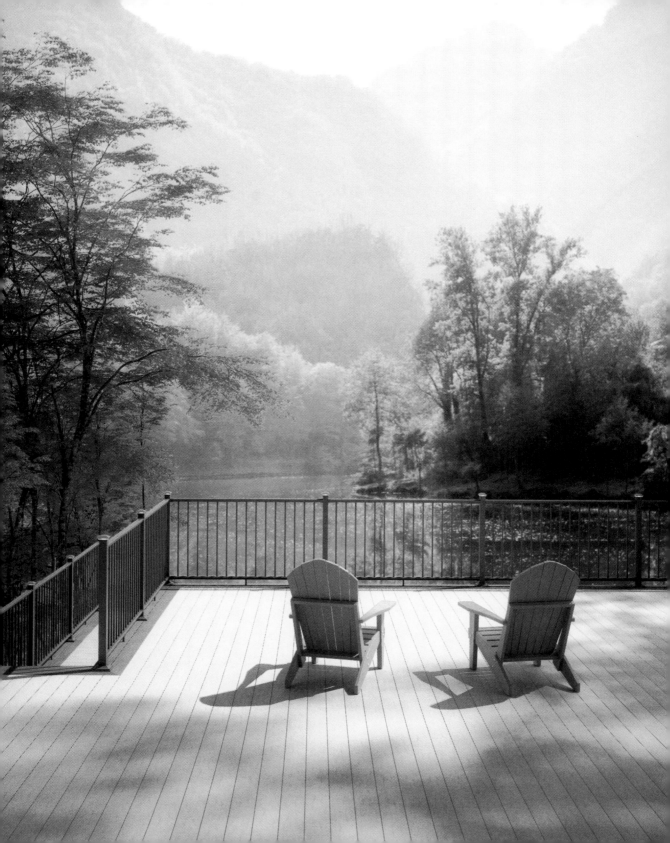

CHECKLISTS & RESOURCES

I s your home as health-enhancing as it can be? Is it safe, accessible, functional, and wellness optimized? Does it support your fitness and longevity? Visit my website—jamiegold .net/wellnessbookextras—for checklists to create your healthiest home (and life!) possible, regardless of whether you rent or own.

You'll also find links there to the Endnotes articles and certification resources for finding healthier products for your living space. These links will be updated as new resources are added to the industry, so you can keep up with the latest offerings.

"Study nature, love nature, stay close to nature. It will never fail you."
—Frank Lloyd Wright (a man who knew something about home design)

ACKNOWLEDGMENTS

Like most great endeavors, books take a team to create, and I've been fortunate with *Wellness by Design* to have some of the best teammates imaginable. These include my Tiller Press/Simon & Schuster colleagues, starting with editor extraordinaire Emily Carleton and including Samantha Lubash, Matthew Michelman, Beth Maglione, Benjamin Holmes, Patrick Sullivan, Matthew Ryan, Michael Anderson, Sam Ford, Marlena Brown, Lauren Ollerhead, and Jennifer Chung. I'm grateful for their willingness to embrace a new concept that straddles design and wellness—how the heck do we categorize this book?—and their skill in bringing it into existence.

I also want to thank these generous friends and colleagues who lent their time and specialized knowledge to ensure that I had the most complete and accurate information possible in their disciplines. These include designers Maria Stapperfenne, Amy Gil, Susan Serra, Patricia Gaylor, Chuck Wheelock, Cheryl Kees Clendenon, Anne Kellett, and Susan Matanguihan; general contractor Sheen Fischer; architect Dean Larkin; technology consultant David VanWert; horticulturalist Mark Davies; personal trainer Lisa Nordquist; and designer/yoga instructor/traditional Chinese medicine doctor Jennifer Ho.

I'm extremely grateful to these health care professionals for their House Call contributions: occupational therapist Brittany Ferri; psychologist Forrest Talley; registered dietitian Martha Lawder; physical therapist Nina Geromel; physicians John La Puma, David Leopold, Jen Trachtenberg, Carrie Lam, and Janette Hope—all MDs; nurse practitioner Maggie Berghoff; and physician's assistant Kristine Blanche.

If you've enjoyed the photos in this book, know that gratitude goes to the dozens of underpaid and overworked communications professionals at design industry brands and associations who sent images from their organizations—sometimes at the eleventh hour—and to the designers who submitted their beautiful wellness-enhancing projects: Lenora DeMars, Suzan Wemlinger, Michala Monroe, Ana Cummings, Diane Foreman, Rafaela Simoes, Laila Colvin, and Kathy Saldana.

I want to thank my athletic community and coaches for helping me stay active and sane during the many months I spent developing and writing this book. You know who you are!

Huge, special thanks go to my literary agent, Steve Harris of CSG Literary Partners, for his exceptional guidance through this publishing venture. And last but definitely not least, I want to thank my own team of professionals: Melissa Kirk, Veronika Miller, Irene Williams, Kim Stebbins, R. Tate Gibson, Andrew Bolsinger, John Atkinson, Ali Rasouly, Barbara Maryott, Heidi Yepis, Debbie Keyler, and Brent Haywood.

Jamie Gold, CKD, CAPS, MCCWC,
San Diego, California

ENDNOTES

CHAPTER 1: WHAT IS WELLNESS DESIGN?

1. Jamie Gold, "Food for Thought #19: In a Chaotic World, Your Home Can Help Reduce Anxiety," Gold Notes: Nuggets from the World of Residential Design, August 28, 2019, https://jamiegold.net/food-for-thought-19-in-a-chaotic-world-your-home-can-help-reduce-anxiety/.

2. Laura Kazmierczak, "Nature's Cure: How Biophilic Design Can Enhance Healing," MCD: Medical Construction & Design, April 18, 2018, https://mcdmag.com/2018/04/natures-cure-how-biophilic-design-can-enhance-healing/#.XfPk4ehKhaR.

CHAPTER 4: SMART HOME TECHNOLOGY

1. Jamie Gold, "Is Your Lighting Making You Sad or Sick?" Forbes.com, January 29, 2019, https://www.forbes.com/sites/jamiegold/2019/01/29/is-your-lighting-making-you-sad-or-sick/#6bb400e06590.

CHAPTER 6: OUTDOOR LIVING SPACES

1. Mihyang An, Stephen M. Colarelli, Kimberly O'Brien, and Melanie E. Boyajian, "Why We Need More Nature at Work: Effects of Natural Elements and Sunlight on Employee Mental Health and Work Attitudes," PLOS One, May 23, 2016, https://journals.plos.org/plosone/article?id=10.1371/journal.pone.0155614.

2. Jane Chertoff, "What Are the Pros and Cons of Saltwater Pools?" Healthline, December 4, 2017, https://www.healthline.com/health/salt-water-pool.

3. Vidushi Kumar, "Five Steps for Cancer-Safe Grilling," American Institute for Cancer Research, June 26, 2018, https://www.aicr.org/press/press-releases/2018/five-steps-for-cancer-safe-grilling.html.

CHAPTER 7: KITCHEN

1. Yvette Brazier, "Is Red Wine Good for You?" Medical News Today, September 7, 2017, https://www.medicalnewstoday.com/articles/265635.php.

2. Robert H. Shmerling, MD, "The Latest Scoop on the Health Benefits of Coffee," *Harvard Health Blog*, Harvard Health Publishing, September 25, 2017, https://www.health.harvard.edu/blog/the-latest-scoop-on-the-health-benefits-of-coffee-2017092512429.

CHAPTER 8: HOME OFFICE/WORKSPACES

1. Edward R. Laskowski, MD, "What are the Risks of Sitting Too Much?" Mayo Clinic, May 8, 2018, https://www.mayoclinic.org/healthy-lifestyle/adult-health/expert-answers/sitting/faq-20058005.

2. "Wrist Rests," OSH Answers Fact Sheets, Canadian Centre for Occupational Health and Safety, July 2, 2015, https://www.ccohs.ca/oshanswers/ergonomics/office/wrist.html.

3. Mayo Clinic Staff, "Office Ergonomics: Your How-to Guide," Mayo Clinic, April 27, 2019, https://www.mayoclinic.org/healthy-lifestyle/adult-health/in-depth/office-ergonomics/art-20046169.

4. Jill Suttie, "Five Ways Music Can Make You Healthier," *Greater Good Magazine*, January 20, 2015, https://greatergood.berkeley.edu/article/item/five_ways_music_can_make_you_healthier.

CHAPTER 9: FITNESS SPACE

1. Cathy Wong, "Types and Benefits of Hydrotherapy," Verywell Health, December 2, 2019, https://www.verywellhealth.com/different-types-of-hydrotherapy-89993.

CHAPTER 11: MASTER BEDROOM

1. Gold, "Is Your Lighting Making You Sad or Sick?"

2. Brandon Peters, MD, "Benefits of Removing the Electronics from the Bedroom," Verywell Health, January 22, 2020, https://www.verywellhealth.com/no-electronics-better-sleep-3014970.

3. "Blue Light Has a Dark Side," Harvard Health Publishing, May 2012 (updated August 13, 2018), https://www.health.harvard.edu/staying-healthy/blue-light-has-a-dark-side.

4. Michelle Drerup, PsyD, "What Is the Ideal Sleeping Temperature for My Bedroom?" Cleveland Clinic, November 8, 2018, https://health.clevelandclinic.org/what-is-the-ideal-sleeping-temperature-for-my-bedroom/.

5. Kristeen Moore and Kristeen Cherney, "Humidifiers and Health," Healthline, April 25, 2017, https://www.healthline.com/health/humidifiers-and-health.

6. Jamie Gold, "Clearing the Indoor Air," *San Diego Union-Tribune*, June 28, 2018, https://www.sandiegouniontribune.com/lifestyle/home-and-garden/sd-hm-indoor-air-20180628-story.html.

CHAPTER 13: KIDS' BEDROOMS

1. Kimberly Coleman-Phox, MPH; Roxana Odouli, MSPH; and De-Kun Li, MD, PhD, "Use of a Fan During Sleep and the Risk of Sudden Infant Death Syndrome," JAMA Network: *JAMA Pediatrics*, October 6, 2008, https://jamanetwork.com/journals/jamapediatrics/fullarticle/380273.

2. "Bunk Bed Safety," American Academy of Pediatrics, https://www.aap.org/en-us/about-the-aap/aap-press-room/aap-press-room-media-center/Pages/Bunk-Bed-Safety.aspx.

CHAPTER 15: GUEST BEDROOM

1. Holly Tiret, "The Benefits Art Therapy Can Have on Mental and Physical Health," Michigan State University: MSU Extension, May 25, 2017, https://www.canr.msu.edu/news/the_benefits_art_therapy_can_have_on_mental_and_physical_health.

PHOTO CREDITS

p. 89:   Photo Courtesy of GelPro Comfort Floor Mats.

p. 91:   Photo Courtesy of Miele.

p. 93:   Photo Courtesy of Bosch home appliances.

p. 99:   Photo Courtesy of Franke Kitchen Systems.

p. 104: Photograph by Ben Sellon for Fully.

p. 107: Photo Courtesy of Herman Miller.

p. 114: Photo Courtesy of Technogym.

p. 117: Photo Courtesy of Designer Ana Cummings, DDA, IDC, CAPS (Owner, ANA Interiors); Photographer: Steve Dutcheshen.

p. 125: Photo Courtesy of Cotto d'Este/Ceramics of Italy member company.

p. 128: Photo Courtesy of Pure Upholstery, division of the Organic Mattress, Inc.

pp. 130–31: Photo Courtesy of Designer Suzan Wemlinger of Suzan J Designs/Photographer: Doug Edmunds.

p. 137: Photo Courtesy of Ponte Giulio, pontegiulio.com.

p. 140: Photo Courtesy of Smith & Noble, smithandnoble.com.

pp. 144–45: Photo Courtesy of M Monroe Design (Interior Design); Photography by Dylan Chandler.

p. 151: Photo Courtesy of Poggenpohl Atlanta—John Coulter, Designer/Brian Gassel Photography.

p. 157: Photo Courtesy of WallDrain from QuickDrain USA.

p. 158: Photo Courtesy of Duravit/Product Designer Phoenix Design.

p. 159: Photo Courtesy of Kohler Co.

p. 167: Photo Courtesy of TOTO.

p. 173: Photo Courtesy of INTER IKEA Systems B.V.

p. 175: Photo Courtesy of 2id Interiors; Designers: R. Simoes, L. Colvin, K. Saldana; Photographer: Emilio Collavino.

p. 178: Photo courtesy of Brizo; Photographer: Gary Sparks Photography, Inc.

p. 184: Photo Courtesy of Smith & Noble, smithandnoble.com.

p. 187: Photo Courtesy of 9 Ten Design. Designer: Lenora DeMars; Photographer: Michael Sage.

p. 194: Photo Courtesy of Designer Diane Foreman, CKBD Allied ASID; Photographer: Roger Turk/Northlight Photography; General Contractor: Neil Kelly Company.

pp. 200–201: Photo Courtesy of LG Electronics USA.

p. 203: Photo Courtesy of BLANCO.

p. 205: Photo Courtesy of Wellborn Cabinet, Inc.

p. 207: Photo Courtesy of BLANCO.

p. 211: Photo Courtesy of INTER IKEA Systems B.V.

p. 213: Photo Courtesy of HandiSOLUTIONS® for Häfele America Co.

p. 218: Photo Courtesy of Deckorators; deckorators.com.

INDEX

porcelain, 29, *30*, 88
quartz, 36, 88, 164
solid surface, 38–39,
88, 164
wood, 30, 31–34, 87
Crock-Pot, 97

D

daybeds, 188
decks, 67–71
decluttering, 10–11, 81
Dekton, 37
dementia, 10
dens, 133–34
desk chairs, 105–6, *107*
desk risers, *104*, 105
digital door locks, 43–44
digital food scales, 97
digital picture frames,
120
digital showers, 50, 165
dimmable lighting, 119,
126, 135, 162
dining chairs, 127
dining rooms, 126–27
dining tables, 126–27
disasters, 14, 24
dishwashers, 95–96, 186
distressed leather
furniture, 129, 134, 135
distressed wood, 134
dog-washing stations,
204, *205*
door locks, digital, 43–44
downdraft vents, 94–95
down pillows and
comforters, 186, 187
drains, linear, 156, *157*
drawer dishwashers,
95–96, 186
drawer locks, biometric,
44, 108
dryers, 198–99
drying racks, 202
drywall, 14, 24
ductless heating and
cooling systems, 212
dust mites, 28, 41, 148,
184, 186
dynamic coefficient of
friction (DCOF), 28,
163

E

elderly. *See* seniors
electrical systems, 19–20
electric fireplaces, 22–23
electric ranges, 101
electronics, bedroom,
142–43, 172
elevators, 124–25
emotional features (of
wellness design), 5–10
Energy Star, 199
engineered stone. *See*
quartz
engineered wood floors,
30–31
en suite bathrooms, 191
entryways, 55–63
front, 55–59, *56–57*
garage, 59
gear management,
62–63
interior, 60–62
mats, 59–60
environmental
protection (smart
technology for), 45–46
Environmental
Protection Agency, 16
ergonomics, 104, 105, 110,
133–34, 203, 204, 216
exercise. *See* fitness;
fitness space

F

falls, 5, 58, 192. *See also*
tripping hazards
family landing zone, 81
Fannie Mae, 11
fans. *See* ceiling fans
farmhouse (apron-front)
sinks, 98
faucets
hands-free, 99–100,
178
kitchen, 99–100
laundry room, 202
voice-controlled, 49
Fenix NTM, 38
Ferri, Brittany, 58, 204
fiberboard, medium-
density, 30, 34–35

fire extinguishers, 5, 101
fireplaces, 22–23, 166
fires, 5, 19, 45, 92, 94, 101
fitness
exercise importance
and benefits, 121
rethinking, x–xi
wellness design
advantages, xii
fitness space, 113–21
dedicated workout
space, 116–19
essentials and extras,
119–20
in garages, 210–12,
211, 217
planning for, 115–16
5G standards, 110
fixtures, smart home,
49–50
flex room. *See* laundry/
flex room
flooring
bamboo, 31, 118, 132
bathroom, 163, 180
bedroom, 170, 184–85
carpeted, 40–41, 132,
134, 170, 184–85
ceramic, 28–30
concrete, sealed, 198
cork, 39, 90, 118, 119
fitness space, 115, 118,
119
kitchen, 89–90
laminate, 118, 132
laundry/flex room,
198
linoleum, 39–40, 90,
118, 119, 134
porcelain, 28–30,
89–90, 180, 198
public living spaces,
132, 134
radiant heat, 29, 48,
164–65, 195
rubber, 40, 118
wood, 30–31, 90, 118,
132, 134, 185
flotation tubs, 166, *167*
fluorescent lighting, 20,
162
fly ash, 40
food processors, 97

pre-drywall inspections, 14
privacy, 51–52, 110, 116
problem-solving and avoidance, 23–25
professional organizers, 210
pro sinks, 99
public living spaces, 123–37
  creating healthier, 123–25
  defined, 123
  dens and studies, 133–34
  dining rooms, 126–27
  game and rec rooms, 134–35
  living rooms and great rooms, 128–33, *130–31*

Q

quartz (engineered stone), 36–38, 88, 98, 164

R

radiant floor heating, 29, 48, 164–65, 195
radiation, 110
radon detectors, 17, 45, 135, 189
recessed lighting, 126
rec room bathrooms, 136, *137*
rec rooms, 134–35
rectified tiles, 163, 198
redwood, 67
refreshers, 199, *200–201*
refrigerators, 95
  mini-, 135, 186, 217
  wine, 96, 135
renters, xiv, 2, 3, 6, 13, 23, 84, 92, 97, 161
resale value of home, 58, 162
resin furniture, 75
respiratory issues, 28, 31, 46, 146
Reye's syndrome, 192

roll-out shelves, 86, 108
roll-out trays, 84–85
rooftop decks, 70
rubber flooring, 40, 118
rugs
  in bedrooms, 185
  outdoor, 70
  in public living spaces, 129, 132, 134

S

safety, 5
  bathroom, 160–61
  kitchen, 101
  nursery, 170–71
  wellness design advantages, xii–xiii
safety data sheet (SDS) (for ceramic and porcelain), 28
saltwater pools, 73
saunas, 165, 166
scalding water, 179. *See also* anti-scald valves
security
  garage, 215
  smart technology for, 43–45
  wellness design advantages, xii–xiii
security lighting, 46
seniors, 5, 28, 34, 51, 58, 127, 132, 179, 185, 192, 204
shades
  automated, 165
  blackout, 141, 185
she sheds, 6
shoe benches, 62
shoes
  removing, 60, 63
  storing, 61–62
shower benches, 156, 193
shower curtains, 179–80
showerheads
  handheld, 155–56, *159*, 179, 193
  with push-button spray mode controls, 193
showers
  digital, 50, 165

in kids' bathrooms, 179–80
outdoor, 74, 164
spa-inspired, 155–57
stand-alone, 155
steam, *18*, 156–57, 162
shower surrounds, 29, 38
shredders, 110
Silestone, 36
sinks
  ceramic, 98
  farmhouse (apron-front), 98
  granite, 98
  integral, 98
  kitchen, 98–100
  laundry room, 202
  porcelain, 98
  pro/workstation/chef, 99
  quartz, 98
  solid surface, 98
  stainless steel, 35, 98
  undermount, 98
sintered stone. *See* porcelain slabs
sitting, disadvantages of, 104–5, 108
sleep, importance of, 139, 140
sleep apnea, 147
sleeper sofas, 188
slip-resistant materials, 5, 28, 29, 70, 89, 115, 163, 180, 192
slow cookers, 97–98
smart home technology, xii–xiii, 43–52
  amenities, 51
  appliances, 48–49
  climate control, 48
  environmental protection, 45–46
  fixtures, 49–50
  hacking, 45, 51
  issues, 51–52
  lighting, 46–47
  security, 43–45
smoke detectors/alarms, 45, 171, 189

well water, 17
wetsuits, proper storage
of, 213
wheelchair users, 94,
95, 124, 155, 185, 186,
193. *See also* mobility
issues
whiteboards, 111, 134,
173
white-noise machines,
143
whole-house water
filtration systems, 19,
162, 180
Wi-Fi-connected
appliances, 198, 215
window coverings
in bathrooms, 141,
180–81

in bedrooms, 140–41,
184, 185
blackout, *140*, 141,
184, 185
windows, opening,
22, 23
wine racks, 96
wine refrigerators, 96,
135
wireless headsets, 110
wood, 67, 87, 90, 118, 132,
185
distressed, 134
engineered, 30–31
uses for, 30–34
wood-burning fireplaces,
22
wool carpeting, 40–41,
170, 185

workstation sinks, 99
wrist rests, 105

Y

yards, 71
yoga, 116, *117*, 118

Z

zinc, 35
zones
enhancements,
84–85
kitchen, 80–86
laundry/flex room,
197
maximizing, 81–83
specialized, 85–86

ABOUT THE AUTHOR

Jamie Gold, CKD, CAPS, MCCWC, is the author of *New Kitchen Ideas That Work* and *New Bathroom Idea Book*, both from Taunton Press. She has worked as a professional kitchen and bathroom designer for sixteen years and is a Mayo Clinic Certified Wellness Coach, consulting on wellness design for homeowners and the building industry. She was named a Top 50 Innovator by leading trade magazine *Kitchen & Bath Design News* in its inaugural list, and has written for *New Home Source*, Forbes.com, and Houzz.

When not working or relaxing at home in her San Diego town house, Jamie can often be found training in the local mountains for her upcoming Kilimanjaro trek.